T0042981

Sugarproof

**Protect Your Family from the
Hidden Dangers of Excess Sugar
with Simple Everyday Fixes**

Michael I. Goran, PhD,
and Emily E. Ventura, PhD, MPH

Avery
an imprint of Penguin Random House
New York

AVERY

an imprint of Penguin Random House LLC
penguinrandomhouse.com

Most Avery books are available at special quantity discounts for bulk purchase
for sales promotions, premiums, fund-raising, and educational needs. Special
books or book excerpts also can be created to fit specific needs. For details, write
SpecialMarkets@penguinrandomhouse.com.

ISBN (hardcover) 9780525541196
ISBN (trade paperback) 9780593421390
ISBN (ebook) 9780525541202

Printed in the United States of America
1st Printing

Book design by Ashley Tucker

CONTENTS

Introduction

I remember the day I decided to write *Sugarproof*. At the time, I was leading a team at the Childhood Obesity Research Center, which I founded at the University of Southern California. For over thirty years, my research has focused on understanding the causes and consequences of obesity in children and how nutrition in early life, even in healthy children, can affect long-term disease risk into adulthood. Over the years, I've seen diet trends come and go, but for me it's all about the data.

On most days, I'm at my desk looking at results from studies involving children who suffer from weight gain and its associated health problems like diabetes, cardiovascular disease, and liver disease. I work to uncover the links between diet and health during infancy and childhood, and then I design and test unique interventions to address these problems. As a nutrition scientist, my hope is always that the raw numbers I love so much will ultimately help us discover how to best prevent the damage that these diseases and disorders do to our children using nutritional approaches. With all sorts of measurement tools like dietary assessments, specific blood tests, MRI scans, body composition measures, and DNA sequencing to test genetic differences and gut microbiome differences, I look for answers through patterns in the data.

But on this day, a different kind of data crossed my desk. What I saw that morning were the results of a laboratory analysis that I'd commissioned, one that looked at products that children love: sweetened beverages, juices, and yogurts. The products I studied included the obvious choices like Coca-Cola, Sprite, and 7UP as well as a broad range of juice drinks popular with kids, including Capri Sun, apple juice, and the orange drink Tampico. The analysis also included snacks and breakfast foods like Go-Gurt and other yogurts, and sweetened breakfast cereals. I knew that these foods and drinks were high in sugar. But I wanted to know more about the different *types* of sugars that might be hidden in them, the ones nutrition labels are not required to disclose. I had a very simple question: *What exactly are in these products that we are routinely feeding to our children?*

The results made my jaw drop. In many cases, the overall amount of sugar in the products was higher than was listed on the food labels. Worse yet, I saw a disturbing amount of hidden fructose in these products. Fructose is a cheap and sweet form of sugar, with many benefits as an ingredient when used in food and beverage production. But unfortunately, more and more research shows that fructose is especially damaging to growing hearts, livers, and brains. I've spent thirty years as a researcher, and long before this day I'd seen sugar do awful things to children. I had researched sugar as a factor in chronic disease, weight gain, and behavioral problems, and I'd become an advocate for families, researching interventions that can help parents rightsize their families' sugar consumption—and that can even turn these diseases around. Even so, this day was a tipping point.

The cold data in front of me led to a visceral understanding: Today's children are not just consuming more sugar than ever before, they're consuming different types of sugar, ones that are uniquely harmful to young bodies—*and their parents don't know it.* Even parents who try to eat healthy don't know what's in their children's food, because it's hidden on the labels, or it's disguised by some other confusing name on the ingredient list. Even parents who are concerned about their child's troublesome symptoms or behaviors don't know that certain types of sugar could be a factor, because most pediatricians themselves often don't know.

Although most of us know that sugar can wreak havoc on adult bodies, many of the parents whose children participate in my research studies are shocked when they hear their child's test results. They simply can't believe it when they find out that their child has dangerously high levels of blood lipids, or that body fat has wrapped itself around their child's internal organs, or that it has even built up inside those organs. Or that sugar might help explain their child's behavioral, emotional, or learning problems. *But he's not overweight,* they say. *But the teacher said her behavior was just a phase. But I ate a lot of sugar when I was a kid, too, and I turned out just fine. But we try to eat healthy at home.* Some parents might curb their own sugar consumption while their children are consuming sweet treats on a daily basis. These parents may believe that kids can eat anything they want and stay healthy as long as they're not overweight. And who can blame them? Big Food has pushed this message for years via commercials and by underwriting studies with a pro-sugar bias. Many parents serve healthy family meals and teach their children to eat well. And *still* dangerous amounts of sugar can sneak into their kids' diets: at snack time, in coffee shops, at sports practices, and through foods that are cleverly labeled and marketed directly to children.

Why is all this so alarming? No matter whether your children are thin or overweight, whether you try to eat healthy family meals or rely on the convenience of fast food, your children are at risk. *All* our kids are at risk. Numerous kinds of sugars and sweeteners have so thoroughly infiltrated our food supply, and food marketing is so insidious, that all our kids can easily consume more sugar than is safe for them. Did you pick up some hormone-free teriyaki chicken and vegetable bowls with sushi at Whole Foods for dinner? This healthy-sounding meal could still have the same amount of added sugar as a can of Coca-Cola. Do you sometimes order pizza on a Friday night? You may not realize, but many pizza companies bake sugar into the dough and use tomato sauce high in added sugars—you'd have to search the fine print of the pizza company's website for the nutrition page, and even *then* you'd need to know enough chemistry to recognize the different sugars that are listed in disguised form, such as malted barley and dextrose. (There are so many different forms of sugar that scientists often refer to these forms in the plural, as "sugars." For ease of communication, we'll stick with the popular term "sugar" in this book, but as you'll learn, there are literally hundreds of sugars on the shelves and in our food products.)

At the same time, science is showing that sugar and sweeteners are major players in the symptoms and disorders that have become increasingly common in our children. Sugar can disrupt the normal growth of internal organs, including the heart, brain, liver, and gut. Despite what you may have heard from studies funded by the sugar industry, the scientific evidence is in, and it is strong. Sugar is linked to all the problems we've listed above. So are sweeteners, which are becoming much more frequently used in foods and drinks marketed to kids. Many common products, such Quaker Chewy Granola Bars, contain both regular sugar *and* low-calorie sweeteners. If your kid is hyper, irritable, moody, or overweight, a diet heavy in sugar or sweeteners could be a reason.

Sugar's damaging effects go even further than anyone might have believed even a few years ago. Our research, and the research of top scientists in the field, has recently shown that sugar has destructive and possibly lasting effects on learning, memory, addictive tendencies, taste preference, appetite regulation, impulse control, and metabolism. And we are learning that growing kids can be much more vulnerable to these effects than adults are. If your children are suffering from learning or behavior problems, or if they can't seem to control what they eat, it's smart to take a close look at their sugar consumption. And sugar goes deeper still, into a child's growing liver and heart. Excess sugar can lead to fatty liver disease, type 2 diabetes, cardiovascular disease, and even an increased risk for some forms of cancer. Those effects can begin before birth, when a mother consumes too much sugar or sugar substitutes, and they continue through breastfeeding, early childhood, and the teenage years. These damaging effects of sugar progress slowly and gradually over time, often with no obvious signs or symptoms, making it difficult to know that underlying diseases are developing.

The news is upsetting, but there is also hope. We can prevent, address, and even in many cases reverse the effects of too much sugar.

That's why, on that day, I decided to continue my investigation into sugars—and to write this book. As a parent, you have the right to know about the effects of different sugars on the growing body from conception through adolescence. While there are many books for adults who want to reduce sugar intake, these books aren't so helpful for families. Not only do they fail to describe how children are uniquely vulnerable to sugar, they don't even try to help parents navigate a world in which sweet foods, snacks, and drinks are constantly marketed to children. I wanted to write this book so that you can see the ways sugar might already be affecting your children. I wanted to write it to provide you with tested and sustainable solutions to protect your kids from their high-sugar food environment.

Because I want you to have a book that is practical as well as science-based, I've joined forces with one of my former graduate students who also worked on my research team for many years, Dr. Emily Ventura. Emily is a former Fulbright scholar and expert in behavioral science, public health nutrition, and recipe development for children and families. She has also led public health campaigns for the Jamie Oliver Food Foundation and Slow Food International. Emily and I have written this book together. We hope that if you have struggled with your difficult symptoms and disorders, searching for solutions and relief, you will find empowerment in these pages. In the first part of this book, you will learn that sugar can be a hidden cause of your child's problems. We'll help you identify the sneaky sources of sugar in your children's diets and discover which sugars are especially harmful, including the array of alternative sweeteners that are now being used more and more often. We'll help you determine whether your children might already be suffering from the effects of too much sugar. In the second part, we'll show you that although sugar is a cause of a host of childhood health problems, it's a cause that you can *do something* about. You can learn to protect your children from a substance that can, invisibly and slowly, literally shorten their lives. Emily and I will draw on our experience as scientists and as parents to show you how to Sugarproof your children—our term for the strategies that protect children from our culture's constant onslaught of sugary temptations. With plans and tools that we have tested in families around the country, along with delicious recipes from Emily in part three, this book will help you rightsize sugar, address the behaviors and problems that could be plaguing your children, and give your kids a healthy new start in life.

—MICHAEL I. GORAN, PHD

A Message from Emily

Like many of you reading this book, I'm a parent. I have two young children, and I'm doing everything I can to feed them nutritious meals and snacks. I also have a PhD in health behavior research and a master's degree in public health. I have taught nutrition to children and families for nearly twenty years. As a mom and a researcher, how do I navigate the sugar-filled, processed-food world our children live in today? I know firsthand that it's not easy.

Being a parent is tough when you know about the real dangers of too much sugar. Because of my work, I know not only that our kids are surrounded by too much sugar and sweeteners but also how easily they can become addicted. But as a parent, I also know that you have to pick your battles. We are all now dealing with challenges like schools that offer chocolate milk, after-school programs that hand out cookies and flavored yogurts as snacks, birthday parties that send our kids home with candy-filled goodie bags, restaurants that serve apple juice with the kids' meals, and grandparents or relatives who show their love with sweets. Do you really want to be *that* parent who constantly says "no"? Do you want your child to feel left out? Do you want to alienate your family?

You may wonder if our focus on reducing sugar is simply a fad, much like the low-fat craze a few decades ago. I was raised in the 1980s and '90s. At that time, the diet and nutrition world told us that we needed to watch how much fat we ate, but there was little talk about sugar. But as manufacturers took out fat from products, they often replaced it with sugar, which is one of the reasons we now have such an issue with sugar and sweeteners in our food supply.

It's clear to me that the root problem in our diet today is our over-reliance on processed foods, which by association means high sugar and/or sweeteners. Seventy percent of processed foods contain sugar. There are so many more prepackaged food options now than there were twenty years ago. Commercial food production companies sweeten many products that you wouldn't normally think of as sweet. The addictive properties of sugars and sweeteners assure that kids—and parents—will want to buy their products again and again. The broadest message I, as a nutritionist and health behavior scientist, could hope to impart is that families should focus on choosing unprocessed foods as much as possible to avoid falling into this addictive trap.

But how can you make this shift in your own household, especially when schedules are hectic and time is limited? As parents, we definitely need to cut ourselves some slack. *Sugarproof* isn't about feeding your kids perfectly, or about avoiding all sugar and processed foods. But ideally you will raise your children to enjoy eating well, and to make good choices even when you are not around. The most effective way to do this, in my experience, is to get kids excited about cooking, which helps them develop a love of fresh fruits and vegetables and other whole foods. I learned many of these concepts in 1998, when I worked as an intern at Alice Waters's Edible Schoolyard Project in Berkeley, California. Working with children to garden and then cook with the fruits and vegetables they grow trained me in this approach and shaped the principles we promote in this book. First and foremost: Simple, unprocessed foods are best.

In *Sugarproof,* we don't want you or your children to see sugar as a villain, but we also don't want to sugarcoat the message (pun intended): Too much of it can be seriously harmful, especially to children. We hope to help allow your kids to enjoy their childhood and youth and some of the sweet treats that come with it—without sabotaging their health. As a parent, I have seen the difference in how my two boys feel and act on days when they have a Sugarproof-style breakfast and stick to our trusty "one treat a day" rule versus how they act on days when we accidentally overdo it with sugar. If you need firsthand evidence that our research is valid, seeing the results in your own children will take your convictions to a whole new level. My hope is that through this book, we can give you the tools to raise children who are healthy, happy, and Sugarproof.

—EMILY VENTURA, PHD, MPH

Part One

This Is Your Child on Sugar

CHAPTER ONE

Growing Up Sweet Can Turn Sour: *All* Our Kids Are at Risk

From the outside, Melissa looked healthy. She was a slender, athletic thirteen-year-old who loved playing basketball and soccer. Yet something was clearly wrong. Despite her long afternoons of sports practice, Melissa had trouble falling asleep. During the night, she woke up multiple times and, because of this, she'd become moody and dark circles emerged under her eyes. On top of everything else, Melissa felt constantly bloated and had frequent stomach cramps.

Under her normal-kid exterior, Melissa's body was silently developing the signs of chronic disease. And behind this disturbing transformation stood one clear factor: the sugar in her diet. Melissa's sugar habits over the course of the day had gradually worked up to a breaking point. She had juice most mornings at breakfast, a cereal bar on school days for a snack, tea sweetened with sugar most evenings, ice cream every other day for dessert at home, and the occasional candy bar from the convenience store down the street from her house when out with friends. Also, Melissa was chewing "sugar-free" Trident gum every day, which is sweetened with a variety of sugar alcohols and other sweeteners.

Melissa doesn't fit what we think of as the profile of a kid on the verge of serious health problems. Melissa wasn't overweight; she wasn't drinking soda; she was physically active; her parents tried to emphasize healthy eating habits. But sugar is now so pervasive, and food marketing so insidious, that during the course of her busy days, Melissa ended up consuming unsafe quantities of not just sugar but also other sweeteners without her parents' full awareness. Because Melissa's parents eventually realized how much sugar Melissa was consuming, they were able to help their daughter reshape her eating habits, and Melissa started to feel energetic and happy again.

Melissa could easily be any child growing up in the United States today. She could be a child in one of our families, or a child in yours. That's exactly the point. No matter whether they are slender or overweight, whether they are active or sedentary, whether they live in a food desert or in a farming community, whether they live in suburbs or cities, *all* our kids are at risk because they are living their lives immersed in sugar. They're at risk for the familiar downsides of sugar—the energy rushes and the crashes. But with our combined fifty years of experience, we know both from our research and from our professional interactions with families that children are at risk for other dangers, too. As a parent, you might attribute symptoms like mood swings, poor sleep, fatigue, difficulty concentrating, or other health issues to stress, hormones, a growth spurt, or an underlying disease. The reality is that all of these problems, whether they seem minor or major, can be connected to too much sugar. Sugar could be causing much more damage to your child's body than you imagined. Compelling new research has shown us that sugar is more dangerous than anyone ever knew, affecting nearly every part of a child's developing body.

The Perfect Sugar Storm

Marco is another kid who seemed pretty healthy from the outside. At age seventeen, he was a big guy. He was overweight, but he was also strong and athletic-looking. And in fact, Marco spent several hours each day playing ball after school and didn't have any other complaints about his health. But underneath his sporty exterior, our evaluation led to a disturbing diagnosis—Marco was very sick.

Because he was overweight, Marco's pediatrician referred him to one of our clinical research studies. Our initial dietary intake uncovered some alarming news. Marco and his family thought he was making reasonable food choices for an active teenager, but in fact he was drinking juice, soda, and a couple of sports drinks every day, which comes to a whopping 100 grams of sugar. That's around 25 teaspoons daily—more than three times the maximum amount we recommend for boys Marco's age. Without realizing it, Marco was delivering a very dangerous sugar load to his liver, more than his body could handle. Part of our study was focused on studying the effects of sugars and excess body weight on liver health in children, so Marco had an MRI of his liver. Marco, his family, and his pediatrician were all stunned to hear the results: Marco was suffering from an extreme case of fatty liver disease, with measurable signs of damage to his liver. If Marco didn't make changes soon, he could eventually find himself in need of a liver transplant.

Fatty liver disease used to be a problem reserved for adult alcoholics. These days, we're no longer surprised when we discover that kids in our clinic are in advanced stages of liver trouble. Not to mention kids with type 2 diabetes or other metabolic disorders. Why? All of us, adults included, are susceptible to the harmful effects from too much sugar. But research shows that children in particular are at *increased* risk. This risk is caused by three critical conditions: kids' inborn preference for sweet flavors; today's high-sugar food environment; and the unique vulnerability of kids' developing bodies to the effects of too much sugar. These three conditions have come together to create a perfect sugar storm for our kids.

Born This Way

How long has it been since you had a package of Pixy Stix? Pop Rocks? Grape Bubble Yum? If you loved these sweets as a kid and have tried them as an adult, you probably wondered how you could ever have enjoyed dumping so much sugar straight into your mouth. But you probably *did* love it when you were a kid. Here's why: Kids have a stronger built-in preference for sweet flavors compared to adults. They are more attracted to both real sugar and low-calorie sweeteners. Given the choice, kids will typically select the sweeter option, and then want more of it. Even amateur scientists have documented the phenomenon. My (Michael's) daughter's elementary school science class performed a simple experiment, asking both kids and teachers to taste five different lemonades of varied sweetness. The younger kids preferred the sweetest version and the teenage kids and adults preferred the less sweet versions.

As your kids have probably informed you, their taste buds really *are* different from yours. Their inborn love of sweet tastes makes evolutionary sense. It ensures that infants will like breast milk, which is sweet. As they start to wean, their preference for sweets helps them avoid bitter-tasting foods that could harm them. A child's love of sweets is not a moral flaw. Kids who clamor for Pixy Stix and Pop Rocks are just being kids. But as you're about to see, this natural attraction to sweetness makes kids highly vulnerable within our modern food environment.

Our Kids Live in a Sugar-Saturated Environment

Alyssa lives in the heart of South Los Angeles and within a food desert—a neighborhood with few options for healthy, fresh food. Alyssa could easily walk to convenience stores and fast-food restaurants from her home and school, but if her family wants to shop at a grocery store that offers produce, they would have to drive twenty minutes or take a long bus ride. Because Alyssa was concerned about her family's history of diabetes, she agreed to participate in our sixteen-week research study, which was designed to help teens eat less sugar. Alyssa shared with us a view of her neighborhood and the impact it had on her food choices: "Right across the street I have the doughnut shop, I have the gas station, the liquor store, and then one block over you have the Burger King, Subway, and another gas station. Another block over you have your Taco Bell/Pizza Hut, and McDonald's. So say . . . I was hungry, and I had about $5 in my pocket, I could either go this way and indulge, and go that way and indulge. Or even go right across the street and get chips and a soda. So either way, it's bad."

Alyssa's situation is extreme, but it's not all that unusual—about 20 percent of all US households are in food deserts. And in some ways, all of us have experiences like hers, whether we live in a true food desert or not. Think about the last time you were in a restaurant, at an airport, on the road, or at a party. You probably had some options for healthy eating, but it's likely that those options were far outnumbered by the junk. Sweets especially tend to dominate: the sweet coffee drinks, sauces, dressings, pastries, and desserts. And as you'll see in a moment, even savory foods often contain sugar as well. What has brought us to this point? Why can't Alyssa escape sugar even when she tries? Why can't you and your kids?

We have some answers to these questions. Five environmental elements contribute to the sugar-loaded food environment in which we now live. Think of them as nutritional weather conditions that children and families have to navigate every day, each contributing to a downpour of sugar (Figure 1):

Figure 1: The Five Environmental Elements Contributing to the Perfect Sugar Storm

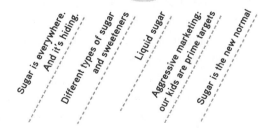

One evening when my (Michael's) daughter was nine, I picked her up from ballet, and she made a special request for turkey dogs for dinner. We stopped at the grocery store, and I ended up doing a bit of research looking for the best choice of hot dog buns. While I checked the nutrition labels, my daughter was rolling her eyes. As the child of a nutrition scientist, she had long ago become used to these types of thorough examinations. As I looked for a decent percentage of whole grains and limited preservatives, I couldn't help but notice that every package on the shelf featured some kind of added sugar. Most of the time, it was listed as the second or third ingredient. The buns that were lowest in sugar had a minimum of 3 or 4 grams of sugar (that's 1 teaspoon) in each bun, so I bought a package of those.

Of course, 1 teaspoon of sugar in a hot dog bun is not really such a big deal. But I was surprised that I couldn't find at least one option without added sugar. And the surprises didn't end there. When we sat down to dinner, none of us would have known the buns contained any sugar. They didn't taste sweet. In fact, they didn't taste very good at all. No one liked them, and we ended up eating the hot dogs without the buns. I couldn't help but wonder: *What would the buns have tasted like without any sugar added?* Of course, as a nutrition scientist, I know that food companies often add sweeteners to mask the taste of other chemicals and preservatives and to enhance palatability. The result can be more of a neutralizing effect than a sweet flavor.

You might fondly recall childhood cultural touchstones like a cone from the ice cream truck, a dripping Popsicle at the swimming pool, or a cookie after school. I grew up in Scotland in the 1960s and '70s, and I have happy memories of the "lemonade van," which came around on Saturday mornings to sell sodas. On occasion, my parents would buy a bottle for the family to share at dinner. For me, it's a happy memory built around ritual, family, and food. We enjoyed it and it is—to this day—a fond memory of childhood. When I recently asked my eighty-four-year-old mother about this, she indicated that there was never any concern about this affecting our health. Soda was a treat to be enjoyed together as a family.

Today, however, sugar is everywhere. It's no longer a treat or saved for a big or special occasion. It's our baseline, our environment, and has become an everyday staple. We've normalized the nearly constant consumption of sugar in childhood. It can seem that everywhere a kid turns, there stands a well-meaning adult offering something temptingly sweet: as an after-school snack, during sports practices, at playdates, or at a grandparent's house. Holidays, traditionally a time to enjoy sweets, have gone supersized. One parent lamented, "It's as if Halloween through Easter has become a six-month-long dessert buffet."

The historical view can provide perspective. During the American colonial period, the amount of sugar consumed by the average person in 1750 was just 4 pounds per year, which is just over 1 teaspoon per day. By 2000, sugar consumption peaked at 150 pounds per year—or a whopping 45 teaspoons per day for the average American. Imagine a 2-pound bag of sugar. In 1750, the average person was consuming two of those bags in a year. By 2000, this increased to one and half bags of sugar each *week*. The United States is now the world's largest per capita consumer of sugar. If you stacked all the sugar as cubes from *one day* of sugar consumption in the United States, it would tower halfway to the moon.

As my encounter with the hot-dog buns shows, it's not just that sugar is offered to kids more often (more about that soon) but that it's *hiding*. Even when you're looking for it, sugar can be hard to spot. Of course it's in cookies, cakes, and ice cream, but it's also in places parents think of as "safe": hot dog buns, bread, granola bars, yogurt, milk, salty snacks, sausages, frozen meals, pasta sauce, salad dressing, and more. Again, a staggering 70 percent of all packaged foods at the grocery store contain some kind of added sugar—for snack foods, the number rises to 80 percent. Sometimes it's easy to read an ingredient list and identify the sugar. When you get in the habit of reading labels, you'll notice how often sugar appears as a first, second, or third ingredient. But there are also whole categories of sugar that are disguised with healthy-sounding names, such as organic brown rice syrup or fruit juice concentrate. And that doesn't even take into account artificial sweeteners like the designed chemicals aspartame, sucralose, and AceK, or all-natural sweeteners like stevia and monk fruit. They may not have the calories, but they can still cause problems for your child's health. In the next chapter, we'll help you identify these hidden forms of sugar so that you can make informed choices for your family. For now, it's enough to recognize that your children are probably consuming vastly more sugar than you did as a kid.

Different Types of Sugar and Sweeteners

Until the 1970s, most sugar was what we'd recognize as plain old white crystalline sugar, known by the chemical name of *sucrose* and extracted from sugarcane or beets. Now, we consume sugar in hundreds of different forms, including high-fructose corn syrup, fruit juice concentrates, and other well-disguised forms of sugar. As food-manufacturing technologies and capacities have expanded, and as a desire for more processed and convenience foods has flourished, so has the expansion of rapidly absorbed, concentrated forms of sugar.

What does this change mean for our kids? The biggest problem is that many of these new types of sugar are higher in fructose than ordinary sugar. In other words, foods and drinks that we used to have growing up were previously sweetened with regular sugar but are now often sweetened with sugars like high-fructose corn syrup or fruit juice concentrates that have a higher proportion of fructose. Over the last century, daily fructose intake in the United States increased from just 12 grams per day to about 75 grams per day. Seventy-five grams per day of *just fructose* is the equivalent of almost 20 teaspoons and accounts for 10 to 12 percent of daily calories for the average adult. As we raise children in this higher-fructose environment, we are starting to see negative effects on their health. Our bodies are simply not designed to tolerate this much fructose, especially in early life. Since fructose is not a natural component of a mother's milk, babies aren't even born with the necessary physiological machinery to handle it. Yet if we compare fructose intake on a per-kilogram basis, infants and children now consume higher amounts than adults. In fact, research has shown that relative to their body weight, infants take in three times as much fructose as teens or adults. As a point of comparison, imagine how a shot of tequila would impact a toddler. An adult weighing 180 pounds can absorb the impact of a shot of alcohol, but the effects on a small child's body would be dramatic. The same goes for fructose: Kids just can't tolerate as much as an adult could. Is it extreme to compare tequila with fructose? No. The human body—especially the liver—processes alcohol and fructose in very similar ways.

In the past couple of decades, we've also seen a rapid increase in different types of alternative sweeteners, or sugar substitutes, that provide sweetness without the calories. These low-calorie sweeteners, or LCS, are now found on every aisle and shelf of the grocery store. Some of these sweeteners are synthetically engineered chemicals like sucralose and aspartame, which are designed to deliver powerful sweetness without the calories, and sugar alcohols, which modify the sugar molecule in a way that retains the sweetness but makes it nonabsorbable. Others may be naturally occurring like stevia (and therefore can be marketed as "all natural"). Children are now being exposed to very high levels of LCS, which can cause their own sets of problems in the human body. These compounds can cause symptoms ranging from acute gastrointestinal distress to long-term effects on the brain, contributing to cognitive decline during later life. And because these sweeteners are so good at mimicking sugar, they fool the brain into thinking they're real. As you'll learn, real sugar can lead to sugar addiction and overeating problems—and because of this trick in the brain, LCS can have the same effect. Most concerning to us is that LCS have not been extensively studied in children.

At the start of this millennium, fewer than 10 percent of American children were consuming LCS in any form on any given day. A decade later, this number had increased to one in four. The main culprit was an increase in the percentage of American children consuming LCS in beverages, such as diet sodas. However, these sweeteners are also widely used in other drinks, foods, condiments, vitamins, and medications with increasing frequency. LCS are often hidden behind factual but deceptive packaging claims, like "no added sugar." And in the case of naturally occurring products such as stevia, labels often say "no artificial sweeteners" or "all-natural ingredients."

Many parents choose the "skinny" or "light" or "all natural" options for kids, believing they're reducing calories and saving their kids from weight gain and future obesity. Sweetness without the calories or the harmful side effects of sugar sounds like an effective combination. However, these sweeteners present a number of potential problems for kids, including changes to developing brains. Worse, many of these products are so new that we just don't have any data about possible side effects or problems they can create for kids as their brains and other internal organs develop and grow.

Liquid Sugar

Kids today, especially young children, are consuming more sugar in liquid form than ever before. A generation ago, kids had only a few options: milk, water, and the occasional juice or soda. Back then, soda was more expensive, less available, and considered a treat. Now kids are drinking more soda than we ever did—but they are also drinking more fruit juice, along with relatively new products such as sports drinks, energy drinks, and blended tea and coffee drinks. All these products deliver high doses of liquid sugar that are very rapidly absorbed and have a more acute effect on the body than sugar eaten in a solid form.

A 2010 study of American toddlers ages twelve to twenty-four months found that added sugar contributed 8.4 percent of their total daily calories; this sugar came mostly from juices and flavored drinks. More than half the toddlers drank fruit juice as their only beverage on any given day. The problem with consuming so much juice is that it changes the types of nutrients kids receive. Their developing bodies, especially their livers, just aren't equipped to handle the sugar load. Many fruit juices and juice drinks contain more sugar and fructose than soda. The numbers for teens are just as alarming. While some statistics now show that overall consumption of sugared soft drinks and juices is on the decline in recent years, the numbers are still much higher now compared to prior generations, and some data shows that consumption is still on the rise in teens.

The generational rise in juice consumption and its potential impact on health was alarming enough for the American Academy of Pediatrics to recommend limits for fruit juice consumption in 2017. The AAP recommended no fruit juice at all before twelve months of age, no more than 4 fluid ounces per day for toddlers (one to three years), 4 to 6 fluid ounces for young children (four to six years), and 8 fluid ounces for children aged seven to eighteen years. This includes all types of fruit juices, even those labeled 100 percent juice and those that are freshly squeezed or pressed at home.

In September 2019, these recommendations were updated in a joint consensus statement released by the Academy of Nutrition and Dietetics, the American Academy of Pediatric Dentistry, the American Academy of Pediatrics, and the American Heart Association. These new recommendations were age-specific. Babies who are newborn to six months old should drink only breast milk or formula. For those six to twelve months old, small amounts of water can be added once solid foods are introduced, but juice should be avoided, as "even 100 percent fruit juice offers no nutritional benefit over whole fruit." For children twelve to twenty-four months old, water is recommended and whole milk can be introduced; in addition, children can drink "a small amount of juice" so long as it's 100 percent juice, "but better yet, serve small pieces of fruit." For children two to five years old, low-fat milk and water are recommended; as for 100 percent fruit juice, "stick to a small amount and remember that adding water can make a little go a long way." The effects of concentrated sugar, especially fructose, in these juices are incredibly negative and can sabotage almost every aspect of childhood development.

Liquid sugar from any source is highly damaging to the body. Compared to sugar that is eaten, the rate of sugar delivery inside the body is much more rapid. Plus, the body has to deal with a large concentration of sugar all at once. Again, fructose is a particular challenge here. The liver has trouble processing large amounts of it when it arrives all at once and in a big dose. The liver is like a kitchen sink garbage disposal. In my (Michael's) house we call the garbage disposal the "gobbler." The gobbler has a bad habit of clogging up the sink, especially when we have guests over. I know I'm not supposed to put carrot or potato peels down the gobbler all at once. If I have a sink full of peels and feed them to the gobbler slowly, then the gobbler works fine. But if I'm in a rush and feed the gobbler a huge pile of peels all at once, the gobbler jams up. The liver behaves in a similar way. Small amounts of fructose, like you'd get from eating a whole, raw apple, are released slowly and do not harm the liver. The fructose is wrapped up inside the fiber, which acts to control its release. But when you drink soda or juice, there is more fructose and it's free in solution without the fiber. In this situation, there is more danger that the liver will get jammed up and the fructose will be converted to fat, which leads to a host of problems.

Despite the problems, we don't rush to judge parents who struggle with beverage choices for their children. One reason for the jump in kids' soda consumption is that processed sweeteners make sugary drinks cheaper than bottled water. And between 1980 and 2010, the relative price of a soda decreased by 35 percent, while the relative price of fruits and vegetables increased by 35 percent. You probably already know that the standard serving sizes for sugary beverages have also increased. In 1955, a cup of Coca-Cola at McDonald's was 7 fluid ounces, whereas today, a children's size Coca-Cola at McDonald's is 12 fluid ounces, and a medium is 21 fluid ounces and costs less than bottled water. Kids can now buy a 44-fluid-ounce soda for 99 cents with free refills. Oftentimes the price is the same no matter the size, so of course kids will choose the biggest one. A 2012 episode of *Parks and Recreation* mocks the trend of wildly increasing soda sizes: The town's restaurant association representative reveals a new child-sized soda, which is an enormous 512 ounces and has to be hefted onto a table with both hands. "It's roughly the size of a two-year-old child," the representative explains brightly.

Aggressive Marketing: Our Kids Are Prime Targets

Sweetness sells. This simple fact is perhaps the main reason that sugar and sweeteners are so pervasive in our food supply. Manufacturers know that sweet foods appeal to children's innate tastes, and they design foods with that preference in mind. These foods begin with the youngest among us: our babies. We live in an environment in which 98 percent of toddlers and 60 percent of infants are consuming added sugars on any given day—because nearly every product designed for their age group is sweetened. Food companies also sweeten infant formula and products intended for post-formula or post-weaning. A recent analysis of 240 of the most popular baby and toddler foods in the United States showed that 100 percent of baby food desserts, 92 percent of fruit snacks, 86 percent of cereal bars, and 57 percent of teething biscuits and cookies contained more than 20 percent of their calories from sugar. Almost 40 percent of all products listed sugar (or some form of sugar) as the first or second ingredient, even those branded as healthy choices. Food companies know that they can begin with babies' desire for sweet foods—and build on it as those babies grow up.

With the sheer number of products that are marketed to kids—and parents—it's hard to make healthy choices. Many parents, including the two of us, have come home from the grocery store with a new product, like a "healthy" yogurt, only to then realize that it is full of sugar (especially when that sugar is hiding under a name that's difficult to spot). Marketers have long known that children are born with a preference for sweet flavors. If they add sugar, they reason, then kids will want to eat their product again and again. Parents tend to assume that the government oversees product labeling with sensible regulations. But food companies have become savvy in disguising sugar in products that we would typically think of as healthy.

The quantity and quality of crops produced in American agriculture today is a testament to technology, yielding vast increases in crops like corn and soybeans. Advances in food chemistry have yielded cheap processed sweeteners like high-fructose corn syrup. The success of the food industry is clear on our crowded supermarket shelves. We are a nation with an excess of beautifully packaged, well-marketed, highly addictive, poor-quality food.

In the 2013 book *Salt Sugar Fat: How the Food Giants Hooked Us*, the Pulitzer Prize–winning journalist Michael Moss introduced the reading public to the "bliss point," the level of sweetness engineered in foods to maximize sales and leave consumers wanting to come back for more. It's the concept food scientists at major companies like Nestlé use when creating a new product. New foods or drinks have to be liked by the majority of a test panel. What's the easiest way to increase likability? Keep adding more sugar until you get enough people to like it. This strategy, and others like it, drives up the level of sugar and sweetness in our food supply.

Companies perfect their recipes, which hook kids and make them want more and more. Then they use age-specific marketing tactics to target their customers directly. Kids see their favorite singers, sports idols, and animated characters promoting candies, snacks, lunch box options, and energy drinks—and they just can't resist. The food and beverage industry spends $10 billion per year advertising to children, including $500 million allotted for sugary drinks alone. Children view around six thousand food commercials per year, mostly for products that are nutrient-poor. Older children and teens are prey to more covert types of marketing, such as Internet ads and product placement in video games. Advertisers are even in schools today, often giving equipment or supplies in exchange for advertising and sales access to students.

Food companies have become very good at targeting groups that are at higher risk of chronic diseases. A recent report from the Rudd Center for Food Policy and Obesity found that in 2017, 86 percent of television advertising on programs targeted to African Americans and 82 percent of ads on programs targeted to Hispanics were focused on junk food, sugary drinks, or other high-sugar snacks and candy. Many of these groups are already at higher risk from the adverse effects of too much sugar. For example, rates of type 2 diabetes are much higher in

Hispanics and African Americans, and fatty liver disease is much higher in Hispanics, so targeting these groups with advertising for sweetened products seems unjust.

Social media and viral fads are the latest ways to get kids to try something new. The nature of gimmicks is that they promote trend-based products, making kids feel left out if they haven't tried the latest new thing. You might remember the Starbucks Unicorn Frappuccino, a sweet, frozen drink festooned with whipped cream and rainbow-colored syrup. When my (Michael's) then ten-year-old daughter bought one with her friends on a school trip and told me about it, I had to look it up on the Starbucks website. The ingredients included a mind-boggling list of added sugars totaling 56 grams—and that was just for the grande, or medium size. That's the equivalent of the sugar in one and a half sodas, or 14 teaspoons, and three times our daily recommendation for added sugar for a fifth grader (not to mention twice the daily recommendation for an adult).

Savvy marketers also target parents, knowing that they are tight on time and sometimes low on patience. Products might feature a tie-in to the latest movie in order to appeal to kids, but they can also feature packaging with phrases like "rich in calcium" or "source of whole grains." Parents often realize that these products have sugar in them but are willing to be guided into the belief that the benefits outweigh potential harms. Kid-friendly products such as sweetened yogurts or flavored milks create a real dilemma for many parents who want to feel good about giving their kids something with calcium, even if it takes some sugar and flavoring to achieve it. Marketers know that parents feel the same way about whole grains and proteins. If their kids are picky eaters, parents usually feel that having them eat *something* is better than having them eat nothing. If that *something* is full of sugar but also includes a few beneficial ingredients, parents feel as if they've scored a win. But between breakfast, lunch box snacks, and packaged convenience foods, the amount of sugar a child consumes each day can quickly add up.

Sugar Is the New Normal

With 70 percent of all foods and 80 percent of snacks for kids containing some kind of sugar, our food and beverage environment has become like a real-life version of the board game Candy Land. But it's not just big industry that's to blame. We parents have adapted to the new, sugary environment, and in most cases, we're the ones who are buying these products. It's hard not to. Parents want to do right by their kids, and most of us want to limit unhealthy foods. At the same time, we pick our battles—and there are a *lot* of battles. While parents know that breakfast is important for children's performance in school, and they want their kids to eat well, the reality is that most of us are short on time in the morning. A healthy breakfast may not go down well or may be rejected. Instead of fighting, parents often serve something sweet and easy, like sweet cereal or frozen waffles with syrup.

And because the environment has changed, there are more opportunities for parents to offer sweets and for kids to be surrounded by sweet offerings in places they like to hang out with friends. For example, coffee shops have been on the rise since the 1980s. They've made good coffee more accessible, and they give everyone a place to meet, talk, and take a break; it's a safe place for kids to hang out with friends or study. But many coffee shops have morphed into sugar dispensaries, creating a situation where kids see the consumption of daily sweet drinks and goodies as normal.

Even if parents try to limit the sugar they give their kids, there are plenty of other well-meaning adults who offer them sweets. What about the elementary school teacher who gives out candy as a reward for turning in homework on time or kind adults who give cookies as gifts? What about all those birthday parties, which feature not just the traditional cake and ice cream but sweet drinks and bags of candy to take home? To make it all harder, kids will naturally resist any parental efforts to curb intake. Try to limit sugar at home or elsewhere and expect to be labeled as "strict" parents, or worse, "mean."

It's not fair that our sugary environment makes it so hard to eat in a way that is reasonable and balanced, but that's our new normal. You're going to need some help, which is why we're here with research, techniques, and recipes that will make it easier. You can get started right away with our Sugar Measuring Activity, which you can find at the end of this chapter. It's an easy and fun way to open your family's eyes to the amount of sugar in everyday products.

Sugar Disrupts Healthy Growth and Development

Yes, kids have an innate preference for sweets. Yes, today's kids are growing up in a sugar-saturated environment. That's bad enough. But the third and final condition of the perfect sugar storm is that sugar can interfere with normal, healthy growth and development. Most of us know that too much sugar isn't healthy for anyone. But as bad as it is for adults, it's even worse for kids. New research shows that too much sugar during critical growth periods puts kids at risk at any age, whether they are still developing in the womb, weaning from breast milk toward solid foods, having a big growth spurt during the elementary years, or going through adolescence.

Dramatic new research shows that their developing bodies are uniquely vulnerable to the effects of too much sugar. In fact, sugar can disrupt the normal growth of the heart, brain, liver, gut, and more. Parents often observe that sugar is linked to their children's wild behavior, hyperactivity, mood disorders, weight gain, acne, and tooth decay—and they are absolutely right. But sugar also enters unexpected territory, with disturbing and possibly lasting effects on learning, memory, addictive tendencies, taste preference, appetite regulation, self-soothing, and metabolism. In clinical studies, we see children like Marco, whose MRIs reveal fat building up not just under the skin but inside vital organs. And we see children whose blood tests reveal high levels of blood lipids or glucose and risk for early diabetes, heart disease, and liver disease. These effects can all be traced back to effects of too much sugar. We know that your child's health is your first priority, so the first part of this book will help you understand just how the sugar they consume affects their behavior, their metabolism, their emotional state, and their success in school (Figure 2).

Figure 2: Effects of Sugar on Kids

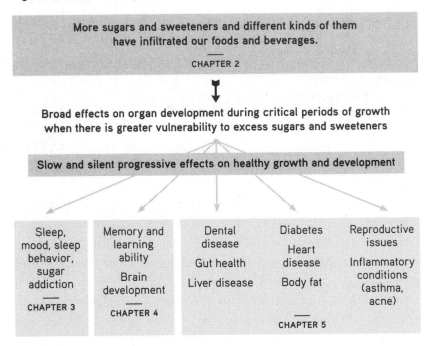

Growing a Sugar Baby

We'd like to emphasize a foundational way that sugar can interrupt health at the very beginning of life. What we call "secondhand sugar" is sugar that is inadvertently transferred to a baby in utero, while nursing, while bottle-feeding, or while eating or drinking foods given by parents or other caregivers. For a fetus or baby, sugar consumption is passive and involuntary, in the same way that smoke inhalation is for a child who sits on the couch next to a parent with a cigarette. Exposure to secondhand sugar can pose a lifelong risk for chronic disease.

When babies are exposed to lots of sweetness (from either real sugar or LCS), their natural preference for sweetness can become even stronger. It's like compound interest. Money grows exponentially in the bank, and under the right conditions, a baby's desire for sugar will grow by leaps and bounds. This process can begin in the womb, where a baby has a continuous feeding line from the placenta through the umbilical cord. If a pregnant mother consumes excessive sugar or sweetness in any form, it can reach the unborn baby, who will then develop an even greater than usual preference for more sweetness. After birth, breast milk is often the sole source of nutrition and sugar. Sugars or sweeteners consumed by a breastfeeding mother can be transmitted to the baby through breast milk. Formula-fed babies often receive additional sugar than nature intended, because some formulas include added sugars beyond the natural lactose found in milk. The exposure to sweetness doesn't end with weaning. Young children are growing, and they need more frequent snacks than adults. Pound for pound, babies, infants, and children eat more frequently throughout the day than the rest of us. If what they're eating is sweet, they're getting more impact from that sweetness. Unfortunately, the brain registers sweet tastes with a desire to eat *more* of that sweetness. Take a baby's innate desire for sweet tastes and couple it with additional exposure to sugar and LCSs through secondhand sugar, and you've got a very young child who is now built to crave—and overeat—sugar. The good news is that even though a sweet taste preference can be shaped in early life, you can also reset it to a lower, more moderate level. We will show you how.

Children's Metabolisms Are Vulnerable to Fructose Early in Life

Studies from my research team were the first to document that fructose from a mother's diet can be transmitted to her baby via breast milk. Physiologically, infants' bodies just aren't designed to be able to tolerate fructose, which is not a natural component of breast milk. Before fructose flooded our food supply, infants who were exclusively breastfed were usually exposed only to lactose (a sugar that naturally occurs in milk), which is broken down into glucose and galactose, smaller sugars that infants can digest and use for energy and growth. There is no fructose in the naturally sourced nutrition of an infant because there isn't *supposed* to be. Now even our youngest children could be exposed to fructose while breastfeeding, if their mothers are drinking or eating it. Of course, when infants are given juice in addition to or instead of breast milk, the problem can be compounded. Infants and little kids just don't have the metabolic machinery to handle fructose, and that in itself can cause digestive issues and set the stage for other problems later in life, such as fatty liver disease and higher risk for things like type 2 diabetes and cardiovascular disease.

Fructose Reprograms Developing Cells

Each of your cells is derived from a stem cell. Stem cells function as a sort of master cell, a cell that hasn't yet formed a special function. As stem cells develop into specialized cells, they can be reprogrammed in the presence of certain nutritional factors—including even very low levels of sugar, especially fructose. For example, exposure to fructose makes it more likely that developing cells will become fat cells. Low-calorie sweeteners, which can mimic many of sugar's effects on the body, have also been shown to reprogram developing cells to become fat cells. Because babies in utero, infants, and children are growing, they are more likely to have a higher number of these developing cells—and once these cells are programmed, they're programmed for a child's entire life. Extra fat cells put a fetus, baby, or young child who is exposed to secondhand sugar at a higher risk of being overweight or obese, which in turn increases the chances of developing a metabolic disorder such as type 2 diabetes.

A Brain Shaped by Sugar

The process of building a mature brain begins in utero and continues through the teenage years. In Chapter 4, "Smarter without Sugar," we'll explain how exposure to too much sugar during periods of development can alter the brain and have irreversible effects on behavior, memory and learning, food preferences, and ability to regulate appetite. In addition, commercials for sweet foods and drinks can activate the brain's reward regions, making kids physiologically more vulnerable to product marketing. It's difficult for most adults to resist sugar marketing, but children, whose executive function is still developing, are even more vulnerable to their effects. In simple terms, this means that the behaviors and traits of children can be shaped irreversibly through exposures and experiences during these critical periods of brain development.

Sugarproof Your Kids

Every day, we all send our kids out into the sugar storm. But there's hope. The purpose of this book is to provide you and your family with simple, realistic, versatile, and sustainable tools to protect your kids from the dangers of too much sugar. When it's hot and sunny, you help your kids apply sunscreen so they can enjoy being outside and not get a sunburn. When it rains, you give them rain boots and a raincoat so they can have fun in the rain and not get soaked. In the same way, kids need protection to brave the elements in our high-sugar food environment. Very young kids need to be protected directly, and older kids can be taught to look after themselves.

In the pages ahead, you'll learn more about the ways sugar might be affecting your kids, and you'll also find tools that help you create new routines and instill healthy habits in your children as they grow. You can keep these tools in your toolkit and come back to them frequently until rightsizing sugar becomes routine and is an acceptable new norm in your house. How you use those tools will change over time as habits change and kids grow. We're not asking you to give up all sugar forever, or to deprive your children from enjoying sweet treats on occasion. We *are* asking you to think about sugar in a whole new way. Our research

Sugar Measuring Activity

It can be hard for kids to understand exactly how much sugar is in their favorite sweet drinks or foods. By doing this activity with your kids, you can help them see exactly how much sugar they are eating and drinking. It can be very revealing even for an adult to see the actual amount of sugar included in sweetened products.

In the first part of the activity, you help your kids learn how to find where sugar is listed on a food label and to understand that this information is listed per serving, not per container. Then you help your kids actually measure out and see how much sugar is in their favorite sweet drinks and foods by using table sugar, a measuring teaspoon, and a plate. Seeing the sugar on a plate makes the message tangible and real so that in the future, kids may give a second thought before choosing an old standby.

Once you complete the activity at home, you may find that it has such an impact that you would like to also lead it with a group of children. We've done this activity at schools and community centers in small groups and even in large lecture settings with audience participation, and it has been very well received by students of all ages and their teachers.

Gather together:

- A bag or large bowl of white table sugar
- A can, bottle, or box of your favorite sugary beverage or food (for example, a soda, juice box, vitamin water, candy bar, cookies, etc.)— anything with a food label that states the amount of sugar.
- A teaspoon
- An empty plate or bowl

1. Take the first item and together as a family take a look at the nutrition label. Note the number of servings in the bottle and the amount of sugar per serving. In the examples shown here, a 12-fluid-ounce can of soda has 1 serving and 39 grams of sugar, a box of apple juice has 1 serving and 22 grams of sugar, a regular hot chocolate has 1 serving and 34 grams of sugar, and a blueberry muffin has 1 serving

and 42 grams of sugar. If there isn't a food label for your favorite item, just ask Google. Note that many bottles (or packages) will have multiple servings, so if your child is used to drinking (or eating) the whole container, then multiply the grams per serving by the number of servings in the container to get the actual amount of sugar (in grams) being consumed.

2. Next apply some simple math. One teaspoon of sugar is 4 grams, so take the total grams of sugar and divide by 4 to get the number of teaspoons. As an example, the 39 grams of sugar in a can of Coca-Cola is 9¾ teaspoons of sugar, or almost 10 teaspoons.

3. Now have your child spoon out the number of teaspoons of sugar in the product (or in one serving of the product if it is a large container/package) from the bag of sugar onto an empty plate or into a bowl.

4. Ask if you'd want to eat that bowl of sugar or put that much sugar on your cereal or in your tea or coffee?

5. Then repeat the above with the other items gathered together to compare them to the first item. Which has the most sugar? Which was most surprising in terms of sugar content?

**Examples of Sugars in Popular Sugary Beverages and Treats.
Spoon It Out to See What It Looks Like!**

12 FL OZ SODA
39g of sugar = 9¾ tsp

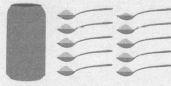

12 FL OZ HOT CHOCOLATE
34g of sugar = 8½ tsp

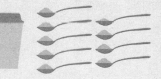

1 BOX OF APPLE JUICE
22g of sugar = 5½ tsp

BLUEBERRY MUFFIN
42g of sugar = 10½ tsp

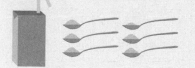

and our firsthand experience tell us that sugar is shortening our kids' lives. In this book, we'll arm you with the information you need to know to protect your kids, and we'll offer you realistic strategies that will make your kids Sugarproof, even in a candy-coated world.

> To view the scientific references cited in this chapter, please visit us online at sugarproofkids.com/bibliography.

CHAPTER TWO

Not All Sugars Are Created Equal: The Many Disguises of Sugar

Two mothers stand on a backyard patio. Behind them, children play and colorful balloons waft about: It's a party. When one mother complains about the red-colored drink on offer, pointing out that it contains high fructose corn syrup, the other one reassures her: "It's made from corn, it's natural, and, like sugar, it's fine in moderation." The first mother is persuaded. She takes a drink and smiles.

This 2008 Corn Refiners Association ad took a beating from the viewing public. One YouTube commentator wryly noted that the same phrasing the ad uses to describe high-fructose corn syrup could apply to cocaine: *It's made from the coca plant, it's natural, and, like other drugs, is fine in moderation.* Yet if you talked to nutrition scientists at the time, many of them would have agreed with the Corn Refiners ad. Not so long ago, it was widely believed that all sugars—including honey, refined cane sugar, raw cane sugar, and high-fructose corn syrup—affected the body in the exact same way. The reasoning: Sugar is harmful because it delivers extra calories that the body doesn't need, and thus contributes to obesity. Therefore, all sugars must be equal. Or are they?

Research has come a long way since then. We now know that all sugars are *not* created equal, because they affect the body in different ways. To make things more complicated, sugar has more than two hundred different names and guises—and that's not counting the growing category of low-calorie sweeteners. In this chapter, we'll help you decode sugar's secret language. We'll reveal some of the science behind each category of sugar and also show you some practical information that you can put to use right away. By the end of this chapter, you'll know how to spot sugar when it's hiding on a label; how different types of sugar are most commonly used; suggested limits for how much sugar your child should eat; and which kinds of sugar are best—and how to avoid some of the worst.

A Sixty-Second History of Sugar

Sugar has been around for thousands of years. The domestication of sugarcane dates back to 8000 BCE, probably originating in New Guinea and spreading to Southeast Asia. But the first real evidence of extracting sugar from plants does not appear until 350 CE, when the process for crystallizing sugar from sugarcane was discovered in India.

Over the next few hundred years, sugar production spread west from India across the Persian Gulf to Middle Eastern countries and later made its way to Europe via the Arab Conquest. By medieval times, sugar consumption had surged among the English nobility and in the royal courts, since sugar and sweet dishes were considered luxury foods fit for people of their lofty stature. There is even historical evidence that King Henry VIII's lavish medieval feasts directly affected his health in the form of gout, which could in part be explained by high sugar consumption.

The average person's diet didn't include much additional sugar until Europeans started to produce sugar themselves. In 1747, Andreas Marggraf, a German chemist, was the first to discover sucrose in beets. By 1813, when Napoleon banned the import of sugar from the British, an alternative European industry had emerged to produce large amounts of sugar on its own, mostly from beets. By 1900, sugar production was well established, which made sugar plentiful, affordable, and an increasingly common part of the average diet. Thanks to the Industrial Revolution, sugar became a food that was widely available to all. As availability surged, so did consumption. Yet sugar remained relatively simple. People added sugar to their food; it tasted good; they added more, and they kept eating.

Figure 3: Some Common Names for Sugar

1. Agave nectar
2. Apple juice concentrate
3. Barbados sugar
4. Barley malt
5. Barley malt syrup
6. Beet sugar
7. Blackstrap molasses
8. Brown rice syrup
9. Brown sugar
10. Buttered syrup
11. Cane juice
12. Cane juice crystals
13. Cane sugar
14. Cane syrup
15. Caramel
16. Carob syrup
17. Castor sugar
18. Coconut nectar
19. Coconut sugar
20. Confectioners' sugar
21. Corn sugar
22. Corn sweetener
23. Corn syrup
24. Corn syrup solids
25. Crystalline fructose
26. Date sugar
27. Dehydrated cane juice
28. Demerara sugar
29. Dextran
30. Dextrose
31. Evaporated cane juice
32. Free-flowing brown sugars
33. Fructose
34. Fruit juice
35. Fruit juice concentrate
36. Galactose
37. Glucose
38. Glucose solids
39. Golden sugar
40. Golden syrup
41. Grape sugar
42. High-fructose corn syrup
43. Honey
44. Icing sugar
45. Invert sugar
46. Jaggery
47. Lactose
48. Malt syrup
49. Maltodextrin
50. Maltol
51. Maltose
52. Malt sugar
53. Mannose
54. Maple syrup
55. Molasses
56. Muscovado
57. Organic agave nectar
58. Organic brown rice syrup
59. Organic cane sugar
60. Organic invert sugar
61. Palm sugar
62. Panela
63. Panocha
64. Pear juice concentrate
65. Piloncillo
66. Powdered sugar
67. Raw sugar
68. Refiner's syrup
69. Rice sugar
70. Rice syrup
71. Saccharose
72. Sorghum syrup
73. Sucanat
74. Sucrose
75. Sugar (granulated)
76. Sweet sorghum
77. Syrup
78. Treacle
79. Trehalose
80. Turbinado sugar
81. Wheat sugar

Today, sugar is no longer so simple. Food technology and science are evolving every day, meaning new kinds of sugar constantly show up on ingredient lists. Marketing techniques are moving fast, too, and it's hard for consumers to keep up. Food and beverage companies often get creative with descriptions, trying to make ingredients sound healthy or to disguise them with complicated names so they don't sound like a sugar. Packaging may say "no artificial sweeteners," "50% less sugar," "refined sugar free," or "fruit-juice sweetened," all of which are phrases that simply mean the product contains some type of sugar or sweetener.

To become an even smarter consumer, you will need to look beyond the marketing claims on products and check ingredient lists for hidden sugar. Figure 3 lists of some of the most common names for sugar. You'll recognize some; others might not even sound like sugar. Some you have not heard of might be lurking in processed foods in your pantry or freezer right now. One way to get your kids interested is to send them on a sugar hunt. Ask them to see how many of the items on the list they can find in your kitchen or at the grocery store.

This list is just the beginning. The Foundation for Eradicating Childhood Obesity has started an online repository for the growing list of names of sugar, and as of March 2020, the list had reached 262 names. As food producers invent new types of sugar or new names, the list grows. You can find the updated version online at http://echoforgood .org/the-added-sugar-repository.

The names for sugar can feel overwhelming. But you don't need to memorize them. When you group them into categories, it's easier to understand how they affect children's bodies and what you can do to make the best choices. Here are the categories we use:

- Sucrose and sucrose-based sugars
- Glucose and glucose-based sugars
- Fructose and fructose-based sugars
- Low-calorie sweeteners

And despite what the old Corn Refiners ad might have you believe, they are not all alike. Not at all. Before we get too deeply immersed in explaining the different sugars, we'd first like to explain some basics. The first thing to know is that if something ends in "-ose," then it's a sugar. The simplest and most common sugars are glucose, fructose, galactose, maltose, sucrose, and lactose. Almost all other sugars are made from or are mixtures of these basic sugars. Glucose, fructose, and galactose are basic sugars and the ones that get absorbed into the body. Sucrose (the most common of all sugars, commonly known as table sugar) is constructed of one glucose molecule connected to one fructose molecule. Lactose (the sugar from milk) is constructed from one glucose molecule connected to one galactose molecule. Maltose is constructed from two glucose molecules connected to each other. These six sugars and their configuration are shown in Figure 4. Although these sugar molecules have very similar chemical makeups, the way they are structured creates differences in the properties of these sugars (for example, taste) and the way they are digested. Some of these differences are also summarized in the figure.

Figure 4: The Basic Building Blocks of All Sugars

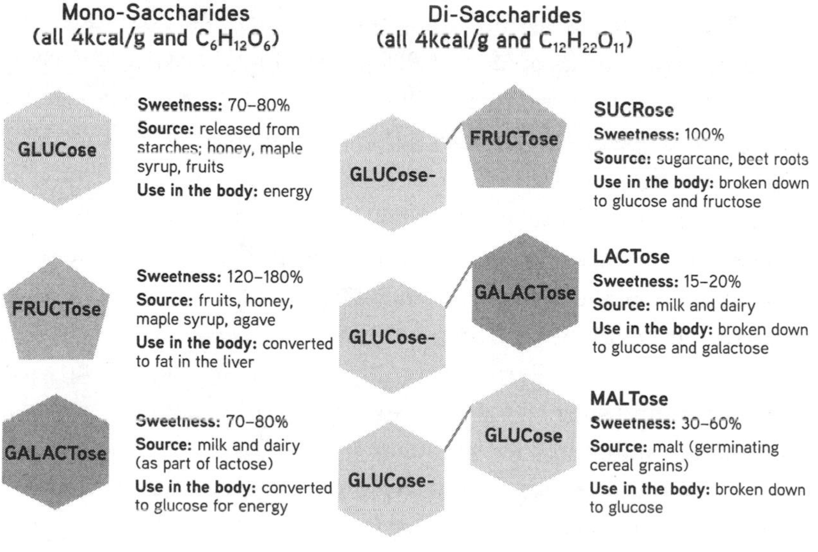

Mono-Saccharides (all 4kcal/g and $C_6H_{12}O_6$)

Di-Saccharides (all 4kcal/g and $C_{12}H_{22}O_{11}$)

GLUCose
Sweetness: 70–80%
Source: released from starches; honey, maple syrup, fruits
Use in the body: energy

FRUCTose
Sweetness: 120–180%
Source: fruits, honey, maple syrup, agave
Use in the body: converted to fat in the liver

GALACTose
Sweetness: 70–80%
Source: milk and dairy (as part of lactose)
Use in the body: converted to glucose for energy

GLUCose– / FRUCTose
SUCRose
Sweetness: 100%
Source: sugarcane, beet roots
Use in the body: broken down to glucose and fructose

GLUCose– GALACTose
LACTose
Sweetness: 15–20%
Source: milk and dairy
Use in the body: broken down to glucose and galactose

GLUCose– / GLUCose
MALTose
Sweetness: 30–60%
Source: malt (germinating cereal grains)
Use in the body: broken down to glucose

These one- and two-part sugars have something important in common. They all produce the same amount of energy, which is measured in calories. They all yield 4 calories of energy per gram of dry weight. One teaspoon of sugar weighs approximately 4 grams, so at 4 calories per gram, there are 16 calories in 1 teaspoon of sugar. This is the same if it's sucrose (table sugar), glucose, or fructose or any other sugar in solid form. Things get a little more complicated when sugars are in liquid form, such as a syrup. The concentrations can vary, which can affect the number of calories per gram, and also how sweet they taste.

All sugars vary in how sweet they taste, which is also summarized in Figure 4. The reference used for measuring sweetness is sucrose—plain table sugar—which is defined as having a sweetness index of 100 percent. Fructose is the sweetest and has a sweetness index of 120 to 180 percent, which means it tastes 20 to 80 percent sweeter than sucrose. Taste is subjective and different people will perceive sweetness differently, so often the sweetness index is given in a range.

Sucrose and Sucrose-Based Sugars

Have you ever opened up a fresh bag of brown sugar, stuck in your nose, and inhaled? It smells so good, with a scent that's rich, almost spicy. And to our modern eyes, brown sugar looks more wholesome and less processed than white sugar does. After all, brown rice is healthier than white rice, and brown bread usually signifies the presence of superior whole grains. But is brown sugar really better than white? Given the choice, should you use brown sugar or raw sugar instead of table sugar to sweeten a batch of breakfast muffins?

We think of white sugar, brown sugar, or raw sugar as classic sugars because, for the most part, they're the products we all grew up with. They're the ingredients you'd find in a home baking pantry or sitting in a little bowl by the coffeemaker. But they are all just essentially different forms of sucrose. Sucrose, the most common sugar, is a white crystalline substance composed of two smaller sugars, glucose and fructose, that are joined together. Sucrose has a slightly more complicated formal name (saccharose), but for our purposes, we'll stick with "sucrose." Sucrose is one of the oldest known sugars and is produced by plants during photosynthesis. Both sugarcane and sugar beets are good at producing sucrose from water and carbon dioxide. For centuries, they've been the main crops grown for sugar production.

To understand how sucrose products are used for different purposes—and why their chemical makeup is nevertheless all the same—it helps to understand sugar production (see Figure 5). Sugar from cane or beets must be extracted from the plant. In the first step of sugar refining, juice is extracted by pressing the sugarcane or sugar beets and adding hot water. This juice is then heated and purified to make cane syrup or beet syrup. The syrup is further heated and evaporated to remove water, producing evaporated cane syrup/juice or evaporated beet syrup/juice. The syrup at this stage is very concentrated, thick, and incredibly sweet.

Figure 5: Types of Sugar Produced from Sugarcane

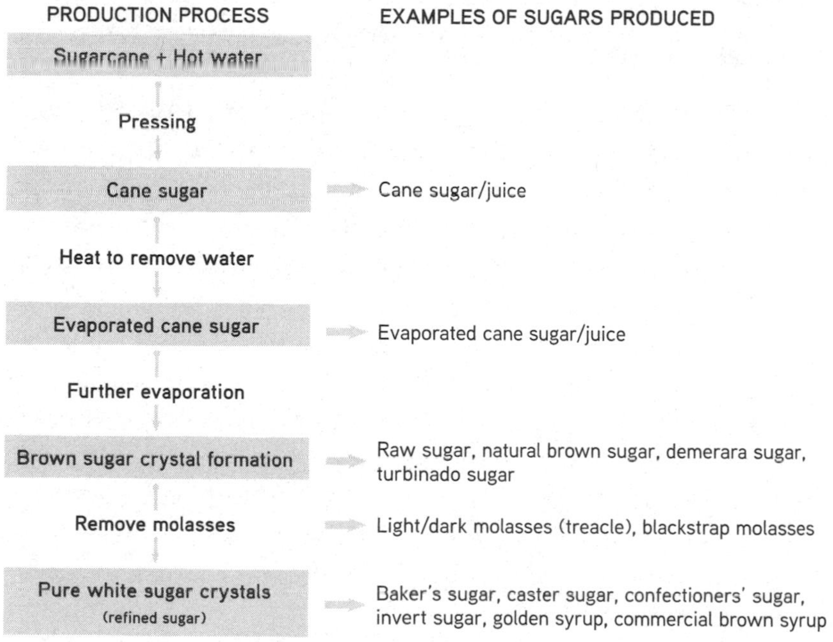

PRODUCTION PROCESS   EXAMPLES OF SUGARS PRODUCED

Sugarcane + Hot water

Pressing

Cane sugar ⟶ Cane sugar/juice

Heat to remove water

Evaporated cane sugar ⟶ Evaporated cane sugar/juice

Further evaporation

Brown sugar crystal formation ⟶ Raw sugar, natural brown sugar, demerara sugar, turbinado sugar

Remove molasses ⟶ Light/dark molasses (treacle), blackstrap molasses

Pure white sugar crystals
(refined sugar) ⟶ Baker's sugar, caster sugar, confectioners' sugar, invert sugar, golden syrup, commercial brown syrup

As the cane or beet juice evaporates, sugar crystals begin to form. At first they're covered in dark liquid molasses. With a spin in a centrifuge, the molasses is separated, and the crystallized sugar begins to look like the sugar we know. Crystallized sugar from beets is white, but sugar crystals that come from sugarcane can still have some molasses content left on them, leaving them brown (referred to as natural brown sugar). These crystals are further washed and processed to make them white and ready for use. Some refiners use animal bone char (cattle bones heated to a very high temperature) for this stage of refining, while others use other charcoal-based filters to remove any residual coloring.

In other words, sugar refining is a long, complicated process. The laborious steps yield sweet sucrose-based products from juice and syrup to crystals of different sizes to by-products like molasses. But all the different types of sugar that are produced along the way possess the exact same chemical composition. They're all still sucrose. And the ways they affect the human body are pretty much the same. When any form of sucrose is ingested, it is quickly broken down into glucose and fructose, which are then absorbed by the body. The glucose is used throughout the body for energy but, as we'll discuss later, the fructose is taken up by the liver where it can be converted to fat.

Brown sugar or raw sugar are not any better for your kids (or you) than white sugar. Nevertheless, it's worth knowing a little about the different forms of sucrose. Many of these sugars are ideal for producing a traditional flavor when baking classic sweet treats. We recognize that certain sweet treats have an important role in our culture and traditions. Our parents and grandparents probably didn't hesitate to serve cakes on birthdays or cookies on holidays—and we shouldn't, either. As long as they are reserved for special occasions, these treats can be a special part of family life. As long as you don't fall into the "every day is a celebration" trap, this is a healthy, appropriate way to consume sugar. Another general rule of thumb that we apply is that if you are making a special treat with any of these forms of sugar, you can use about half of what is called for in a typical recipe. It doesn't affect the texture, and the taste is often sweet enough.

Here are some of the most common forms of the sucrose family, along with their uses. They're all considered refined sugar:

Granulated sugar: Everyday white table sugar. This is the most common form of sucrose with granulated crystals and is commonly used in baking and cooking. When you bake a birthday cake, you probably use granulated sugar.

Superfine, caster, or baker's sugar: The same as table sugar, except the crystals are more finely grained. It dissolves easily and is thus useful in adding to cold drinks.

Powdered, confectioners', or icing sugar: This sugar is finely ground until it becomes powdery and may also contain a small amount of anti-caking agent, such as cornstarch. Often used in frostings.

Decorating or sanding sugar: Another common form of sucrose, these coarse crystals are larger than regular granulated sugar. Think of the green- and red-colored sugar crystals that are often sprinkled over holiday cookies.

Commercial brown sugar: Brown sugar that is produced by adding molasses (see below) back to refined white sugar from cane or beets. This way, the amount of molasses can be kept consistent and controlled so that the sugar reaches a desired degree of brownness. This soft sugar is often used in cookies.

Caramel: Caramel is made by slowly heating sucrose and turning it into an amber-colored, thick syrup. In the heating process, the sugar molecules break down and then re-form into a variety of compounds that provide different color and flavor profiles.

Invert sugar: In the case of invert sugar, the sucrose is treated with acid and/or heat to break the sucrose molecule down to its components of glucose and fructose to make a syrup. This is useful for some recipes because it does not crystallize as easily. One commercial form of invert sugar is golden syrup, which is popular in the UK.

The following sugars are produced during the intermediate stages of the sucrose production process. Some of these forms of unrefined sugar may be perceived as healthier, since they are less processed and thus closer to their natural state. Don't be fooled. With the exception of molasses, they all have exactly the same chemical composition as regular table sugar:

Evaporated cane juice: The exact sugar content of evaporated cane juice or evaporated beet juice depends on how concentrated the solution is. This sugar often appears on ingredient labels, probably because it sounds healthy. But it's really just partially refined regular sugar. In 2012, the yogurt maker Chobani was sued for claiming its yogurt had no added sugar, when in fact it contained evaporated cane juice. This case remains unresolved.

Demerara, turbinado, or "raw" sugar: All of these products are less refined or less processed than pure white sugar. While they have a slightly more complex flavor profile than white sugar due to the hint of molasses, they do not offer significant nutritional benefits.

Molasses: Molasses is the dark liquid separated from the sugar crystals using a centrifuge after the boiling process. Since some sucrose hasn't crystallized, molasses still tastes sweet and can be used to add flavor and sweetness to recipes. While both sugarcane and sugar beet refining processes produce molasses, only molasses made from sugarcane is fit for human consumption. (Molasses made from beets is used for livestock and—surprise— is mixed with salt to de-ice roads.) Light molasses is produced from the first extraction, or spinning, of the centrifuge, and has a mild taste and a higher sugar content. Dark molasses is made by further boiling the light molasses so that more sugar is extracted, leaving a darker syrup with a stronger taste. If the syrup is boiled for a third time and even more sugar is removed, it leaves behind a thicker, bitter, and less sweet molasses known as blackstrap molasses. All types of molasses are a source of calcium, iron, magnesium, and manganese, but there are plenty of superior dietary sources for these minerals. Molasses is used to add a deep flavor to baked goods such as gingerbread.

Natural brown sugar: Sugar that still contains some molasses, which makes it stickier and darker in color. This is often used in cookies or added to oatmeal.

Muscovado sugar: Made by grinding unrefined cane sugar that still contains molasses, resulting in a very dark brown sugar. Muscovado sugar has become popular for baking as well as adding to savory dishes for depth of flavor.

Other unrefined sugars: Additional unrefined brown sugars are also popular in many Asian and South American countries and cuisines. These sugars include panocha, piloncillo, and panela. Made from cane juice, they're generated in varying stages of the production process and are often sold in bricks or cones.

When it comes to sucrose-based sugars, keep in mind that whether they are brown or white, solid or liquid, derived from sugarcane or sugar beet, the chemical composition of the sugar is the same. Whether it's the white sugar you choose at the coffee shop or the brown sugar you sprinkle over oatmeal, they are all the same form of sucrose. You might prefer one flavor over another, or a slightly less processed version, but the nutritional differences are minimal.

Glucose and Glucose-Based Sugars: The Sugar That's Hard to Spot

You've probably seen things like dextrin and maltodextrin on food labels. Did you know that these substances are all sugars made from glucose? What about corn syrup, brown rice syrup, or barley malt extract? These are also sugars from the glucose family, and their names make them especially tricky to spot.

Glucose is a very social molecule that likes to get together with other glucose molecules to form other sugars and starches. When there are more than ten glucose molecules in a chain, this structure becomes more of a starch than a sugar. Starches found in corn, wheat, potatoes, rice, and oats are essentially composed of long, branched chains of glucose molecules that are all joined together. Starches are how plants store their energy, often encased with fiber, and we cultivate these starches for our own food. They are broken down during digestion to yield glucose, which is then used for energy around the body.

From a biological perspective, glucose is the most important sugar. It is the main form of sugar that circulates in blood and the one that provides energy to all parts of the body. All cells in the body require energy to work, and that energy comes from glucose. Because of its critical need for energy, the body carefully regulates the amount of glucose in the blood using the hormone insulin. The best sources of glucose are whole grains or complex carbohydrates because in this case the glucose is released slowly over time and becomes easier to regulate to avoid high spikes or sudden drops in blood glucose levels.

Even though glucose is of vital importance to the body, typical sources found in products on grocery store shelves (such as corn syrup) or as added sugars in foods are not ideal sources of energy. Glucose sugars are often highly concentrated and rapidly broken down, raising your blood sugar quickly. And they tend to appear in products that aren't wholesome foods, as we'll see below. Some of the most common forms of glucose are hard to identify on labels because their names don't sound like other sugars:

Dextrose: Just another name for glucose, dextrose is typically produced from corn and is chemically identical to glucose. Manufacturers often use it as a sweetener in foods and drinks ranging from granola bars to cereals to sauces to drinks such as Gatorade.

Maltose or malt sugar: Maltose is composed of two glucose molecules connected to each other and is naturally found in malted (fermented) cereal grains and in some fruits and vegetables like sweet potatoes. It is about half as sweet as sucrose, and you'll often see it added as a sweetener in bread and cereal products, hard candies, and frozen desserts. A similar sugar is maltotriose, which is composed of three glucose molecules joined together. When consumed, these sugars rapidly break down to glucose to be used for energy.

Trehalose (also known as mycose or tremalose): Trehalose is very similar to maltose, but its two glucose molecules are joined together in a different way that makes the sugar more stable, even at high temperatures. It is used most often in frozen foods and as an additive to ice cream because it lowers the freezing point and makes it easier to scoop. Unfortunately, trehalose could lead to unintended health problems beyond those normally caused by sugar. A study published in 2018 found that certain strains of the bacteria *Clostridium difficile* thrive on trehalose and cause intestinal distress. *Clostridium difficile* is a bacteria normally found in our intestine, but when this gut bacteria feeds on trehalose (as happens when we eat foods that contain it), it can evolve into a more dangerous strain that can cause major GI disruption. This sugar was introduced into the food supply around the year 2000, and soon after, doctors saw a sudden increase in *C. diff* infection.

Maltodextrin: A partially broken-down starch consisting of anywhere from three to seventeen molecules of glucose joined together in a chain, maltodextrin blurs the line between a sugar and starch, but we generally consider it a sugar since its molecules are more easily digested than most starches and cause a quick release of glucose in the body. In the United States, maltodextrin is typically made from corn, but it can also be made from wheat (or any starch) and is cheap to produce. Maltodextrin is used in food production as a thickener more than a sweetener; you can find it in infant formulas, instant puddings, sauces, dressings, and seasonings.

Dextrin: Very similar to maltodextrin, dextrin typically consists of more than twenty glucose molecules joined together, so technically it is a starch. Dextrin is used as a thickener and is rapidly broken down during digestion into glucose.

Corn syrup: Not to be confused with high-fructose corn syrup, corn syrup is made by mashing corn into a starch and then breaking down that starch to release the sugars, forming a concentrated glucose solution. Corn syrup, also called glucose syrup, is 100 percent glucose. You'll also see light corn syrup products that are flavored with vanilla, or dark corn syrups with added molasses.

Rice syrup and brown rice syrup: Made by cooking rice and then adding enzymes to break the starch down into sugars—mainly maltose, maltotriose, and some glucose—and then reducing the liquid down to a syrup. It is used with increasing frequency in products like energy bars, cereals, and even infant formula. For example, the first ingredient in a Clif Bar is "organic brown rice syrup." Rice-based syrups, high in glucose, release glucose into the bloodstream very rapidly, making them popular for bars and gel products advertising an energy boost for activity.

Barley malt syrup or extract: A sweetener with a thick consistency similar to molasses, with a malt-like flavor. It's about half as sweet as sucrose.

Manufacturers know that most parents don't realize that these substances are sugar. Sometimes they use glucose-based sugars to slide sugar into products that you probably don't think of as sweet, such as frozen foods, salad dressing, or highly processed foods. But these hidden sugars can add up quickly in a child's diet and they won't even be enjoying "sugary" treats.

Fructose: The Confusing Sugar

Have you ever seen a Freestyle soda machine in a fast-food restaurant or at the movies? These brightly colored machines feature a touch screen and the ability to dispense 165 different sodas. Kids love the Freestyle. They like the choices, they like pushing on the screen, and they love mixing the options to make their own customized flavor. But here's the real secret of their appeal: The sodas they dispense are ultra potent, with a higher formulation of high fructose corn syrup than regular soda in a can . And when it comes to sugar, fructose can be one of the most hazardous.

Fructose is probably the most confusing and misunderstood of all sugars, and it can also be the worst for kids. Fructose has the same chemical makeup as glucose, but its shape is different. Glucose is hexagonal, but the backbone of the fructose molecule is arranged in a pentagon. This difference drastically alters the properties of fructose and the way it is handled in the body. For starters, your body can't use fructose as a direct source of energy. That's because the liver takes up almost all the fructose that we consume, especially when we consume it in high amounts, which is exactly what we get when we drink juice or sugary soda. And in the liver, fructose is converted to fat. This newly synthesized fat can build up in the liver—which is exactly what happened to Marco, the high school athlete who drank multiple sweet beverages every day and developed fatty liver disease. Additionally, the newly synthesized fat gets released and transported around the body. This contributes to lipid buildup in the blood, which in turn leads to heart disease. If you remember nothing else about the dangers of too much fructose, remember this: *The liver turns fructose into fat.*

Why isn't this danger of fructose more widely understood? One reason is that it's associated with fruit, so it sounds healthy. It's true that whole fruit contains fructose, along with glucose and many favorable nutrients like fiber. The precise sugar profile of fruit depends on the kind of fruit, the variety, and the ripeness—but when you eat a piece of fruit, you don't need to worry. In whole fruit, the fructose is encased in a fiber-rich flesh that slows and reduces its absorption in the body and its metabolism in the liver. This whole package creates a slow-release system for fructose, easing it into your bloodstream and protecting you from its negative effects. Fructose usually becomes problematic only when it is consumed in concentrated or liquid forms, such as in soda, apple or orange juice, and other sugar-sweetened beverages. When a lot of fructose gets consumed and absorbed rapidly, without the fiber to slow its absorption, it goes rapidly and directly to the liver for conversion into fat. When consumed in lower amounts, some of the fructose can be converted to glucose and the effect on the liver isn't as severe.

Another way that fructose is different from glucose is that it tastes twice as sweet. What could be bad about having more sweetness with less volume? Plenty. Since fructose is much sweeter than any of the other sugars, food producers are drawn to it. For them, fructose offers a bigger bang for the buck. This makes fructose a popular added sugar in products like yogurt and beverages like Vitamin Water, sodas, and sports drinks—which in turn means that our kids are downing this sugar in quantities and in ways that nature never imagined. Their livers are taking in fructose at high speeds, without the whole-food packaging of real fruit to slow things down.

High-Fructose Corn Syrup: The Industrial Mixed Sweetener

Let's talk about the elephant in the sugar bowl: high-fructose corn syrup (HFCS). One of the most notorious of sweeteners, HFCS does not occur anywhere in nature; it is a synthetic sweetener that can be made only in a factory. It is produced from corn, is a mixture of glucose and fructose, and is now ubiquitous in our food supply.

How did HFCS enter our food supply? Politics and economics were the prime factors. In 1957, two American chemists, Richard Marshall and Earl Kooi, discovered a method for converting the glucose in corn syrup to fructose. In 1971, Japanese scientists figured out a mass production process for this conversion. The timing was perfect. HFCS turned out to be an ideal solution for the rising food prices, food shortages, and the unpredictable availability of imported sugar that occurred in the 1970s. The US government helped carve out a secure market for HFCS by making changes to the Farm Bill, with incentives to corn farmers to grow larger quantities of corn to produce processed products like HFCS. In 1977, Congress imposed new taxes and limits on sugar imports to protect American sugar producers from foreign competition. The result of these policies was to drive the price of sugar up and the price of industrialized sweeteners like HFCS down. By the late 1970s and early 1980s, corn production soared, and so did the production and use of HFCS.

In 1984, the nation's two largest beverage manufacturers—Pepsi and Coca-Cola—replaced sugar with HFCS in their soft drinks. By 1995, HFCS had eclipsed sugar as the dominant sweetener in our food supply. In 1980, Americans consumed just three million tons of HFCS, which increased to eight million tons in 1995, and then decreased slightly in 2017 to about seven million tons. As other countries began using HFCS—in Europe it's known as "iso-glucose"—global consumption increased as well.

HFCS is a manufacturer's dream. It's cheaper and sweeter than regular sugar. It can be synthesized in mass quantities from an abundant and cheap source of corn. Once produced, HFCS is already a liquid, so it's more efficient in beverage production. It remains shelf-stable through extremes in temperature. When used in baked goods, HFCS produces a perfectly tempting and consistent color and a pleasing texture, what experts call "mouth feel." And when products with HFCS are frozen, the HFCS causes a reduced freezing point, which keeps products soft or even pourable. With all of these attractive qualities, what's not to love?

The food and beverage industry has long maintained that HFCS is almost identical to sucrose, with only two subtle differences. According to the industry, one of the two differences is that in HFCS, the fructose and glucose are already separated whereas in sucrose they are joined together. No argument there. And second, the industry says that any extra fructose in HFCS is negligible.

We heard about those claims, but we weren't convinced. As nutrition scientists studying how kids' diets affect their health, we kept running into a wall. We wanted to know exactly how much fructose is in products sweetened with HFCS, but we couldn't get the information. Food labels and food databases don't contain details about fructose, and companies don't release it. We wanted to know how much fructose kids were consuming, and that's when we decided to conduct our lab analysis of sweetened products that kids love. The results of the first study, published in 2011, and then verified in three different independent laboratories in 2014, sparked a controversy.

In regular sugar (sucrose), there is an equal number of fructose and glucose molecules. But we found that in the five most popular HFCS-sweetened sodas (Coca-Cola, Pepsi, Dr Pepper, Mountain Dew, and Sprite), the sugar was a mix of 60 percent fructose and 40 percent glucose. Remember, the industry had not revealed this information. We had to investigate this for ourselves. This difference in percentage might seem trivial, but in reality this small difference can have significant effects on the body. For the HFCS-sweetened sodas, this translates to three molecules of fructose for every two glucose molecules, or

50 percent more fructose than glucose. That's 50 percent more fructose that will be released into kids' livers, turned into fat, and sent back into the bloodstream.

How do we explain this discrepancy? Food companies are not required by law to disclose the exact amount of fructose relative to glucose in the HFCS they use. However, the most common form of HFCS used to make beverages is called HFCS-55, which is made up of 55 percent fructose, 42 percent glucose, and 3 percent other sugars. Other forms of HFCS include HFCS-42, HFCS-65, and even HFCS-90, meaning it contains 90 percent fructose. Because labeling laws only require a company to list HFCS as an ingredient, consumers aren't privy to which formula or how much is used in any given product, so as consumers, we don't really know how much fructose we are consuming.

Our study results prompted some important questions. We wondered why there would be 60 percent fructose in the drinks if manufacturers claimed they used HFCS-55. One possibility is that the HFCS-55 was actually blended with some HFCS-90, leading to a higher fructose concentration. The FDA guidelines approved HFCS-55 as a safe ingredient; it required a "minimum" of 55 percent fructose and allowed for the unrestricted sales and use of the more concentrated HFCS-90. The form of HFCS does not need to be disclosed on food labels.

Additional research has shown that the proportion of fructose is important. In one human study, forty adult volunteers were asked to drink two different varieties of Dr Pepper in random order. One was made with regular sugar and the other was made with HFCS. Blood samples were collected from the volunteers over a period of six hours. Results showed that during that time, there was 20 percent more fructose circulating in the blood of the participants who'd consumed the HFCS soda. The group consuming the HFCS version also showed significantly elevated blood pressure, as well as other risk markers for diabetes and cardiovascular disease, along with increased uric acid, which is a by-product of fructose metabolism and contributes to inflammation and gout.

Natural Sugars Containing High Levels of Fructose

Many parents we talk to are worried about their kids' sugar consumption and turn to natural sugars like agave. They might buy treats that contain these sugars or use them to make homemade cakes, muffins, or cookies for their kids, and it feels like a win-win. Their kids get the sweet flavors they love, and the parents feel that they've found a healthy workaround. But these well-intentioned parents, who try to avoid serving their kids HFCS, are possibly baking high levels of fructose right into their kids' foods. Some natural-sounding sweeteners are even higher in fructose than HFCS. Here's a rundown:

Agave syrup or nectar: Agave syrup is made by heating the juice that is extracted from the leaves of the agave plant. The exact composition of the sugars depends on the species of agave used, but it can be as high as 90 percent fructose. That's astounding. Some people will tell you that the advantage of agave syrup is that it's usually so sweet that you don't need to add much. But even if you use it in small amounts over time, the amount of fructose quickly adds up. Because of its high percentage of fructose, we don't recommend using agave.

Fruit juice concentrates: These popular commercial sweeteners are made from any fruit juice that is boiled until much of the water evaporates and it forms a syrup. Apple, pear, and grape juices are the most popular, but any fruit can be concentrated and used as an additive sweetener. Manufacturers often use a combination of fruits, and the exact contents may or may not be disclosed on the food label. When you see the term "fruit juice concentrate," you're looking at a food product sweetened with the concentrated syrup produced from a generic and unknown mixture of fruits. While these sugars do not exclusively contain fructose, they do contain a high amount. For example, apple and pear juice concentrates are about 70 percent fructose and 30 percent glucose (that's more fructose than in soda made with HFCS), whereas grape juice and orange juice concentrate contain fructose in the 40 to 50 percent range. There is often no fiber in these juices to slow the rise in blood sugar, although in some cases small amounts of soluble fiber might be retained in the juice. Were you hoping that the presence of vitamin C makes fruit juice concentrates nutritious? Sorry. The production process also damages the vitamin C from the juice, making it unusable to the body. Avoid products made with fruit juice concentrates whenever possible, as they are often high in fructose.

Fruit sugar: When fruit juice concentrates are further evaporated into a crystallized form, the result is fruit sugar. With names like organic grape sugar, fruit sugar, or crystalline fructose, these fruit-based sugars may sound healthier, but they aren't. While we don't know exactly how much fructose is in these products (except for crystalline fructose, which is purified 100 percent fructose), we do know that they are similar to fruit juice concentrates. These sugars are of huge benefit to food companies, which can advertise products containing them with such labels as "fruit juice sweetened," "contains real fruit," "no sugar added," and "all natural ingredients." There is really no nutritional benefit to fruit sugars. In fact, they may be more problematic than sucrose because fruit sugar can be much higher in fructose.

Natural Sugars with Lower Fructose

These natural products do contain fructose, but in lower amounts, and the fructose is balanced by other kinds of sugar molecules or other nutrients. They have a slightly higher nutritional value than other forms of sugar, and sometimes they contain small amounts of fiber, which would allow the sugar to release slowly into the body instead of all at once. Also, these natural sugars tend to have a more complex flavor profile. Remember, though, they are still sugar—and American kids are eating too much sugar in any form:

Maple syrup: Maple syrup is made from the sap of maple trees. Pure maple syrup is mostly sucrose with smaller amounts of free glucose and fructose, but the sugar profile varies and can depend on the grade. Typically, maple syrup includes fructose and glucose in equal amounts, which means that it's nutritionally similar to table sugar. Maple syrup has a more complex flavor profile, and you may end up using less of it than you would ordinary sugar. It also contains small amounts of minerals like calcium, potassium, iron, and manganese. Beware of maple-flavored pancake syrups, which are not derived from maple trees and often contain high fructose corn syrup.

Sweet sorghum, sorghum syrup, and sorghum molasses: These syrups are made from the stalk of the sorghum plant. Once the stalk is pressed and boiled, sorghum yields a sweet syrup with a high sugar content. These products have been traditionally produced and consumed in the southern United States, but they are becoming increasingly popular worldwide. Like maple syrup, sorghum syrup contains mostly sucrose, with smaller amounts of glucose and fructose. It also contains small amounts of vitamins and minerals, including vitamin B_6, manganese, and potassium, though you have to consume a lot to get these benefits. It tastes similar to molasses but with a slightly sour flavor.

Honey: Honey has been used for a long time for both food and medicine and was perhaps the first sweetener used by humans. Made by bees from plant nectar, it consists of mostly fructose (30 to 45 percent by weight) and glucose (25 to 40 percent by weight), with the rest made up of maltose, sucrose, and other sugars. The exact mixture of these sugars is highly variable and in some cases can have almost twice as much fructose as glucose. Honey also has very modest amounts of vitamins, including vitamin C and vitamins B_6 and B_2 (riboflavin) and other complex sugars and therefore may have slight nutritional advantages. It's important to note, however, that honey is not recommended for infants (under age one), because it may contain bacteria that their bodies are not yet able to handle.

Palm sugar and coconut sugar: These sugars are extracted from the sap of palm trees, including coconut and date palms. Palm sugars have a long history in Southeast Asia and the Pacific Rim regions and are called a variety of different names, including jaggery. Both are about 70 to 80 percent sucrose; the rest is mostly a mixture of glucose and fructose. You may hear these products referred to as "healthier." Because they go through a less rigorous refinement process, they do have some slight nutritional advantages over white sugar, with more micronutrients and a small amount of fiber called inulin.

Date sugar: This sugar is made by finely grinding dehydrated dates, with the advantage of retaining other nutrients found in the whole fruit (which include fiber, vitamins, and minerals). The precise sugar composition depends on the variety of dates used, but typically date sugar has a mix of fructose and glucose, sometimes with a smaller amount of sucrose. Since date sugar is not 100 percent sugar, there are fewer calories per teaspoon, and its small amount of fiber helps slow the rise in blood sugar. Of course, its nutritional advantages do not magically make this sugar a healthy food. You still need to use it with discrimination.

Date syrup: This is made by boiling dates with water and then blending or pressing them. Some of the fiber from the dates may be removed during the process of turning them into a syrup, but some fiber remains, which helps slow the rise in blood sugar. Like date sugar, it can be healthier than sucrose, but you still need to use it sparingly.

Take the Clif Bar Challenge

Look at these ingredients from the nutrition label of a Clif Bar (Blueberry Crisp Flavor). Test your knowledge by identifying which items are a form of sugar. If that's easy for you, try identifying the ingredients that are high in fructose:

Organic Brown Rice Syrup, Organic Rolled Oats, Soy Protein Isolate, Organic Roasted Soybeans, Organic Cane Syrup, Rice Flour, Organic Almonds, Concentrated Apple Puree, Organic Soy Flour, Organic Oat Fiber, Dried Blueberries, Organic High Oleic Sunflower Oil, Organic Invert Sugar Syrup, Apple Juice Concentrate, Organic Glucose Syrup, Blueberry Puree, Sea Salt, Natural Flavors, Barley Malt Extract, Citric Acid, Pectin, Elderberry Juice Concentrate (for Color), Lemon Powder, Mixed Tocopherols (Antioxidant).

Answers appear at the end of the chapter.

The Healthiest Source of Sugar: Whole Fruit

"What's the healthiest sugar to use in baking and treats?"

"Is there any way my kids can sweeten their oatmeal without adding sugar?"

We love hearing questions like these, because they're good questions. And we have a good answer: In general, the best way to sweeten is with a naturally sweet whole fruit such as a banana, apple, or pear, or with unsweetened dried fruit like dates, raisins, or figs. The Sugarproof recipes that you'll find in the back of this book use these foods as sweeteners in pancakes, muffins, cakes, granola, and more. Each variety of whole fruit has a different chemical composition, but they all contain some fructose. Yes, fructose. As you now know, fructose can be harmful when it is isolated, concentrated, and ingested in large quantities—but when it's packaged as nature intended, inside a banana or an apple, it is both sweet and safe in moderate amounts. Whole fruits provide sweetness along with natural phytochemicals and vitamins that enhance the nutritional value of a food. They are good sources of fiber, which helps slow the digestion of glucose and fructose and are less likely to cause spikes in your child's blood sugar.

From Sucralose to Stevia: Low-Calorie Sweeteners

Up to now, we've focused on real sugar—sugar that, for better or worse, provides calories for energy. However, a growing category of sugar substitutes presents its own set of issues and questions. These sugar substitutes are sometimes called nonnutritive sweeteners or high-intensity sweeteners. We refer to them as low-calorie sweeteners (LCS). LCS are the sweeteners found in the ubiquitous pink, blue, and yellow packets found alongside the sugar in cafés and restaurants. Some have been around for a long time, such as saccharin (Sweet'N Low; pink packets), aspartame (Equal; blue packets), or sucralose (Splenda; yellow packets). There are also newer natural options like stevia, monk fruit, and allulose.

The taste of LCS is as much as hundreds or even tens of thousands times sweeter than sugar. This intensely sweet taste can be delivered either with fewer calories or no calories at all; most are completely calorie-free. In addition, LCS are often mixed and blended into other products simply to offset any unfavorable properties, such as a bitter aftertaste.

When LCS first came on the market, they were considered a nutritional breakthrough: sweetness without calories. This fueled growth of a whole new market of diet sodas and reduced-calorie foods that did not compromise sweetness. The idea was that diabetic consumers, dieters, and others could enjoy a wide range of beverages, cookies, and candies without sugar. Some folks will tell you that by removing the calories, LCS avoids the harmful effects delivered by too much sugar, such as excess weight gain or the effects of fructose on the liver. However, new research is showing LCS can contribute their own separate set of effects on the body.

How do these products sweeten without real sugar? In order for us to register a sweet taste, sugar molecules need to have a specific shape. That shape turns on special receptors in the tongue and mouth. These sensors are uniquely shaped protein molecules with sockets that are perfectly shaped so that sugar molecules can plug into them. Think of these receptors as a lock and the sugar molecules as the key that fits to open the lock. If the key is the right fit, then the lock opens and the receptor sends a signal from the mouth to the brain. Both sugar and LCS molecules fit the lock. When a sugar or an LCS molecule slides into the receptor socket, it activates a signal that the brain reads as SWEET TASTE. The better the fit of the molecule into the receptor, the stronger the signal to the brain and the stronger the perception of sweet taste. This fit explains why, for example, fructose registers in the brain as much sweeter than glucose. The fructose molecule is shaped differently, giving it a better fit in the receptor. Some LCS have been intentionally engineered to powerfully stimulate these sweet receptors even at very low concentrations.

These alternative sugars might seem like a simple solution to reducing the sugar in your children's diet, but they illustrate perfectly why you should think about the effects of sugar that go beyond their calorie content and effects on body weight. Among other problems, sugar creates a vicious circle: Eat something sweet, and you'll want more of it. Keep eating enough of it, and sugar can harm internal organs. Low-calorie sweeteners appear to have the same effect. They do save calories, but they don't circumvent the bigger problems of sugar addiction, overeating, and potential organ damage. Also, it turns out there are sweet taste receptors not just in the mouth but also in other parts of the body, such as the gut and the pancreas. When LCS are consumed, they can activate these other receptors in the same way as if they were triggered by real sugar. For example, if the body thinks it is sensing sugar through these receptors, then it will produce insulin to make sure this "sugar" is taken up into different organs to be used for energy. This will then result in an uptake of sugar from the bloodstream when it is not really needed, and trigger hunger sensations to replace that sugar with more. Long story, short . . . blood sugar falls and as a result we are driven to eat more food.

Most of these alternative sugars are processed very differently by the body compared to real sugar. In some cases, they are broken down into other compounds that can be harmful—and in other cases they are not broken down at all and can affect gut health. We also don't have enough information about LCS to understand their long-term effects on children's growth and development. In addition, because of the proliferation of LCS in food products and the lax labeling requirements, consumers have a difficult time spotting them. You will need to look out for them on ingredient lists. Some of the newer ones are so powerfully strong that only trace amounts need to be added. The amount needed can be so small that it does not even need to be listed as an ingredient at all.

Figure 6: List of Names for Low- or Non-Calorie Sweeteners

1. Acesulfame K (AceK)
2. Advantame
3. Allulose
4. Aspartame (Equal)
5. Cyclamate
6. Erythritol
7. Lactilol
8. Malitol
9. Mannitol
10. Monk Fruit
11. Neotame
12. Saccharin (Sweet N' Low)
13. Stevia
14. Sucralose (Splenda)
15. Truvia (Rebaudioside A)
16. Sorbitol
17. Xylitol
18. Yacon Syrup

No Added Sugar? Think Again.

Maybe you were shopping for things to pack for your kids' school lunches and bought a new, healthy-looking yogurt or a drink that was advertised as "no added sugar" and the nutrition labels indicated 0 grams of sugar. Maybe you later took a second look at the label and noticed that it contained aspartame or sucralose or stevia. The label was technically correct—these substances are not sugar—but you probably didn't intend to buy a product that had been sweetened. It's an easy mistake to make. One of the leading experts in consumption patterns of LCS is Allison Sylvetsky Meni, an assistant professor of nutrition at Georgetown University. She shared with us that she had recently become hooked on a new brand of almonds ("Vanilla Roast"), whose label trumpeted "No Artificial Ingredients." It was only later when she went back to buy another pack that she noticed that they contained stevia. Since stevia is a naturally occurring sweetener, the label was technically accurate. Without careful review at the time of purchase, even an expert missed the added sweetener.

Additionally, artificial and "natural" LCS are also found in a variety of unlabeled sources like children's vitamins and medicines. Food and beverage companies are required to list all ingredients, so labels should note if an LCS is used, but there is no requirement to specify the actual amount in any given food or beverage.

Low-Calorie Sweeteners Your Kids Might Be Consuming

Would it surprise you to know that the first low-calorie sweetener was discovered by the Romans? They would take grape juice, boil it down in lead pots, and then use the concentrate, known as *sapa*, as a sweetener. Unfortunately, this process also led to a reaction between the lead in the pots and the sugars from the grapes, producing lead acetate. It has a sweet taste, so there was no way the Romans could have known that their sapa was also toxic and likely caused lead poisoning.

Flash forward two thousand years. Now we have a wide variety of LCS with different chemical structures, effects on the body, taste perception, and sensory properties. Like the Romans, we are ingesting substances that we may not fully understand—and that could carry hidden dangers. We *especially* need a lot more information about the long-term effects of LCS on growing bodies.

As a parent, you need at least a passing acquaintance with the most common LCS. Parents who would never dream of giving their child a Diet Coke often have no idea that the same alternative sweeteners used in diet sodas appear alongside regular sugar in everyday products, including ones that are designed to appeal to kids, such as juice drinks and yogurts. Since the turn of the millennium, children's consumption of these alternative sweeteners has increased dramatically. The most recent estimates show that 25 percent of children consume products with alternative sweeteners. But with a little more information, you can spot and avoid LCS. Below is a rundown of those you might know and those that are not as familiar-sounding, like sorbitol, which can be found in many kids' lunch bags as an ingredient in some popular soft granola bars. Low-calorie sweeteners can be broken down into three categories: artificial sweeteners, sugar alcohols, and natural sweeteners.

Artificial Sweeteners

When you think of sweeteners, you probably think of these products. New sweeteners are undergoing regulatory approval every day, and these artificially created compounds sometimes bear no chemical resemblance to sugar molecules. They are much sweeter than sucrose and can be used in very small amounts as sweeteners. Each has a different chemical composition, and each has different effects on the human body:

AceK (sold as Sunett and Sweet One): AceK is 200 times sweeter than sucrose and has a faster onset of sweetness than sucrose but also a slightly bitter aftertaste and therefore is often used in conjunction with other sweeteners like sucralose or aspartame. Since it's stable at high temperatures, you can find it in processed baked goods. AceK can seem harmless because it is not broken down by the body and is excreted in urine. But AceK binds to sweet taste receptors in the mouth *and* in other parts of the body such as in the gut and in the brain, where it can have some of the same damaging effects as regular sugars.

Aspartame (sold as Equal; blue packets): Aspartame is 200 times sweeter than sucrose and induces a long-lasting taste that can linger on the palate annoyingly, so it is often mixed and used in conjunction with AceK. Aspartame is not technically a low-calorie sweetener because when it's broken down, it still yields the same energy as sucrose: 4 calories per gram. However, because it is so sweet, manufacturers need to add only a very small amount to get the desired sweet taste. Much like AceK, it binds to sweet taste receptors in the mouth, gut, and brain—and it is also broken down during digestion to produce chemicals that you would not want in your child's body, including methanol, formaldehyde, and formic acid, albeit at low levels below toxic thresholds. Since the breakdown of aspartame also includes production of phenylalanine, aspartame can't be used by people with phenylketonuria, a metabolism disorder known as PKU.

Advantame (no trade name): This molecule is derived from aspartame and is the most recent LCS to be approved by the FDA (2014). Advantame is twenty thousand to forty thousand times sweeter than sucrose. Because it is so sweet, only trace amounts need to be added to achieve required sweetness. For example, only one thousandth of a gram of advantame is all that is required to achieve the same amount of sweetness as sugar in a can of soda. Because it's used in such trace amounts, it is unclear if advantame even needs to be named specifically on the ingredient list or just included under a generic listing of "artificial flavor." The manufacturer's website lists one of the major benefits of advantame as "requires no special labeling."

Neotame (trade name NutraSweet Neotame): Neotame is ten thousand times sweeter than sucrose and is very similar to aspartame, but because it's around fifty times sweeter, it can be used in much lower amounts. Even trace amounts of this compound are sufficient to add sweetness; like advantame, it might not even appear on ingredient lists. Neotame is rapidly broken down inside the body into alarming by-products (aspartic acid, methanol, formaldehyde, and formic acid). One small advantage of neotame is that the aspartame molecule is modified in a way that blocks the release of phenylalanine, so people with PKU can use it. But no specific studies of neotame have been conducted in humans, let alone in young children, so no one knows how safe it is.

Saccharin (trade name Sweet'N Low; pink packets): Saccharin is three hundred times sweeter than sucrose, has no calories, and is mostly excreted by the body unchanged in urine. It has a bitter or metallic aftertaste and is therefore often used in combination with other sweeteners, usually aspartame. Studies in the 1970s showed that lab rats fed saccharin experienced increased rates of bladder cancer, but later studies concluded that this danger is unique to rats because of certain properties of male rat urine. However, there's a different reason to be concerned: Studies in animals and humans have shown that saccharin can disrupt the natural balance of the gut microbiome, which can then affect other health outcomes such as risk for type 2 diabetes. Saccharin is now the third most widely used LCS in the United States after sucralose and aspartame. It is heat stable, so it can be found in baked goods.

Sucralose (trade name Splenda; yellow packets): The most commonly used sweetener in the United States, sucralose is three hundred to a thousand times sweeter than regular sugar. It is made by adding chlorine molecules to sucrose, producing, in effect, *chlorinated* sugar. By itself it has zero calories, but it's often used with fillers like dextrose or maltodextrin that can add 2 to 4 calories per teaspoon. It tends to taste a little better than other sweeteners. Its sweet flavor comes on about as quickly as sugar's does, and it lasts longer. Like many other artificial sweeteners, it's used in processed baked goods. Sucralose is not absorbed or digested; it is excreted in the stool, which means that it might alter gut bacteria.

Cyclamate (sold as Sugar Twin): Cyclamate is thirty to fifty times sweeter than table sugar and often used in combination with other sweeteners to balance tastes. It is stable under heat, so again, you might find it on the label of processed baked goods. Cyclamate was banned for use in the United States in 1970 due to studies showing increased cases of bladder cancer. However, it is still approved in other countries around the world, including Canada and the EU.

Sugar Alcohols

While these sweeteners are closely related to the chemical structure of sugar molecules, they've been modified so that they retain sweetness but aren't absorbed and therefore provide fewer than 4 calories per gram—and sometimes *no* calories at all. Sugar alcohols like xylitol are used widely in products like low-calorie chewing gum to replace sugar, and they are also being used in more foods and beverages.

Sugar alcohols are often used in combination with other sweeteners to increase sweetness. Sugar alcohols can also be used in baking and candy-making because they crystallize just like sugar. Since sugar alcohols don't affect blood sugar levels, you'll see them in popular low-calorie chocolates and candy often marketed to diabetics. They're not an ideal substitute, since they don't caramelize the way sugar does and therefore do not provide the same flavor profile. Additionally, many consumers report gastrointestinal side effects, such as bloating.

When you're looking at ingredient lists, keep your eyes open for xylitol, sorbitol, lactitol, and mannitol. They're all forms of sugar alcohols. You might also see erythritol, which is becoming more widely used and is a little different from the other sugar alcohols. It has 60 to 80 percent of the sweetness as regular sugar, but only negligible amounts are absorbed by the body for energy, allowing it to provide only 0.2 calories per grams and to have a negligible effect on blood glucose levels.

Erythritol is often used in combination with stevia to increase sweetness and to mimic the mouthfeel of regular sugar; by itself, erythritol gives a cooling mint-like effect in the mouth, which is balanced by the stevia. You can find this stevia/erythritol combination in popular brands like Halo Top low-calorie ice cream or the Bai line of low-calorie beverages. This combination of substances has developed a following, but we can't recommend it because, like other LCS, we don't know much about how it affects children's growth and development.

Natural Sweeteners

Several LCS products carry the labels "all natural" or "no artificial sweeteners." It's not a lie. They're all made from naturally occurring plant compounds. Consumers tend to feel better about buying them, because they're not chemicals created in a laboratory. But because we do not know enough about them, we do not recommend any of these products at this time:

> **Stevia and rebaodioside (trade names Truvia, Pure Via, Stevia in the Raw):** Stevia is a naturally occurring sweetener extracted from the leaves of the stevia plant, which some cultures have long used to sweeten drinks. The extracts of the leaf are rich in compounds called *steviol glycosides*, which can be 150 to 300 times sweeter than regular sugar. Stevia and rebaodioside—another extract from the plant—are heat stable so they can be used in baking even though they don't crystallize in the same way sugar does.
>
> The sweet taste of stevia tends to have a slower onset and longer duration than sucrose, and some stevia products have a bitter aftertaste, so you may see other sweeteners used in conjunction with it. The brand sold as Truvia, for example, also contains erythritol and other flavor enhancers. Coca-Cola Life, the green-labeled soda you may have seen in grocery stores, is made with a mixture of cane sugar and stevia leaf extract and contains only 60 percent of the sugar in regular Coca-Cola. Other companies like Sanpellegrino are beginning to use stevia in sparkling

sodas to reduce the amount of regular sugar they use. Stevia is not absorbed by the body, so it may have effects in the gut, such as altering its microbiome.

Monk fruit, also known as luo han guo (sold as Monk Fruit in the Raw and PureLo): Monk fruit is native to Southern China and looks like a small green melon or gourd. It's used as a traditional sweetener in many Southeast Asian cultures. In 1995, Proctor & Gamble patented a process for extracting the sweetener and removing offending flavors. The extract from monk fruit is three hundred times sweeter than sugar, thanks to a group of compounds known as mogrosides. This sweetener has zero calories and does not affect blood sugar levels, but some people report an unpleasant aftertaste. Monk fruit is available for sale in powdered form in the baking aisle, and it is increasingly being used to sweeten beverages as well as foods like ice cream.

Yacon syrup: Extracted from the roots of the yacon plant that grows in the Andes Mountains, this syrup has traditionally been used in South America for medicinal purposes. However, it's now growing in popularity as an LCS. Yacon syrup contains a high amount of a type of fiber called fructooligosaccharides (FOS), which may be helpful for promoting a healthy gut. But beware. FOS is composed of many fructose molecules joined together in a chain and, when consumed, they can be partially digested, releasing fructose, which gets absorbed and then has the same effects on the body as if it were from any other source of fructose.

Allulose and tagatose: Both allulose and tagatose are rare sugars. Rare sugars are found in nature in figs, raisins, maple syrup, and brown sugar, for example—but in very small amounts. These sugars have similar sweetness to table sugar but are not metabolized by the body and instead are just excreted in urine. Allulose is a white granular substance and can be made to look and feel just like sucrose with 70 percent of the sweetness. This gives it many of the same cooking and baking properties, including crystallization in candy, chocolates, and ice cream. The chemical structure of allulose is very similar to that of fructose and glucose; however, subtle differences in its molecular arrangement make it stable in the body so that it is not broken down for energy. Initial studies, though limited at this time, show that allulose does not affect blood sugar levels and can improve glucose control and weight loss. For all these reasons, allulose is rapidly gaining in popularity.

Tagatose is very similar to allulose. It's found in milk and some fruits in low amounts with about 90 percent of the sweetness of table sugar and about a third of the calories. Tagatose also does not affect blood glucose or insulin levels.

Although the properties of these emerging sweeteners are certainly appealing to manufacturers, we do not yet know if they are safe for long-term use. They have not been rigorously studied, and we do not know much about their health effects, especially in children.

Are LCS Safe for Children?

We hear this question a lot. The simple answer is that we don't really know much about their long-term effects—and that is enough for us to recommend that you avoid them.

Here is what we do know, and it's not much. The FDA has approved some LCS under the category of "generally recognized as safe" (known as GRAS) for use below an acceptable daily intake. Most of these acceptable daily intake levels are actually quite high and unlikely to be reached by any child. In order to hit the upper limit of the intake level, a two-year-old would have to consume the same amount of aspartame or AceK contained in four or five diet sodas. A teenager would have to consume the equivalent of twenty diet sodas. But the GRAS levels for other LCS are more attainable. For example, a toddler who drinks more than one diet soda containing saccharin or sucralose a day would exceed the daily maximum. So would a teen who drinks four or five. But what is *really* important to keep in mind is that these limits don't tell us a whole lot about a product's overall safety. The FDA sets these levels based on amounts that have the potential to cause cancer or mutations. A GRAS approval usually means that a product has not caused cancer in lab studies of animals. But what about other, longer-term effects, such as alteration of taste preferences, diabetes, obesity (thanks to those altered taste preferences), or disruption of gut microbiomes? If an LCS were to cause these effects, the amount needed to cause problems would likely be much lower. In addition, infants and children do not have fully developed guts or kidneys. They might not be able to clear these products from the body in the same way that adults do—and no one knows what kinds of problems could result.

Several leading health organizations have made recommendations for the use of LCS in the general population, but none have been specific to children. The American Diabetes Association (ADA), Canadian Diabetes Association, American Heart Association (AHA), and the US Academy of Nutrition and Dietetics have all released endorsements for the use of LCS, but these statements have been very vague, and they acknowledge that we cannot be certain about the long-term effects of these alternatives. For example, in a joint statement in 2012, the ADA and the AHA said there was not enough data to make a conclusive determination of whether the use of LCS was beneficial for adults for managing obesity or related issues like heart disease or diabetes. None of these recommendations have been specific for children or pregnant women. The most recent 2015 USDA Dietary Guidelines for Americans concluded that LCS should *not* be used as a sugar substitute because of lack of information about long-term effects.

Because of this uncertainty, our recommendation for LCS is very simple: We do not endorse their use for children in any way. This may change as we learn more, but the appropriately rigorous studies will take time. Low-calorie sweeteners are not proven to be safe for children, and even the naturally occurring ones should be avoided. We also do not suggest LCS use in pregnancy or nursing, given that LCS can cross the placenta, may affect the developing baby, and even can pass through to the infant via breast milk. If you want to be extra sure to avoid LCS in any processed foods, then try to buy organic products because synthetic sweeteners cannot be added to an organic product; otherwise it would lose its organic label.

We hope that one day more will be known about the long-term effects of the many different kinds of LCS on children. At that point, it will be possible to give recommendations that are specific to each product. Until then, a good way to Sugarproof your children is to avoid all LCS.

Food Labels and Sugar Content

Food labels can seem overwhelming and difficult to read, but once you know a few tricks, they are easy to navigate. US food labels are in the process of changing and will be required to list not just the total grams of sugar in a product but also the grams of *added sugar*, making evaluating sugar content much easier. Larger food companies are already implementing the changes, which were required to be in place by January 2020. Smaller food companies will have until January 2021 to make the switch. Single-ingredient products like honey and maple syrup aren't required to switch until July 2021. For a while, consumers will see both the old and the new food labels in circulation. The figure below compares the original and new food labels side by side.

There are a few elements to note. First, serving size is more prominent in the new labels. The package may look small or you might be used to eating it as a single serving, but there may be two or even three servings. The label will specify the size of the serving. When in doubt, measure it to see how it really looks. Regardless if it's one serving or eight in a package, the nutrition facts are always based on one serving. If you plan to eat or drink the whole container, you will need to multiply the grams of sugar listed by the number of servings in the container. For example, if there are two servings of juice in a bottle and the total sugars listed are 20 grams or 5 teaspoons per serving, then you will need to multiply 20x2 to get the total sugars in the container, which would be 40 grams or 10 teaspoons.

Figure 7: The US Nutrition Facts label (left) compared to the new format introduced in 2020

Old Label

Nutrition Facts
Serving Size 2/3 cup (55g)
Servings Per Container About 8

Amount Per Serving

Calories 230   Calories from Fat 72

% Daily Value*

Total Fat 8g	**12%**
Saturated Fat 1g	**5%**
Trans Fat 0g	
Cholesterol 0mg	**0%**
Sodium 160mg	**7%**
Total Carbohydrate 37g	**12%**
Dietary Fiber 4g	**16%**
Sugars 12g	
Protein 3g	

Vitamin A	10%
Vitamin C	8*
Calcium	20%
Iron	45%

* Percent Daily Values are based on a 2,000 calorie diet. Your daily value may be higher or lower depending on your calorie needs.

		Calories:	2,000	2,500
Total Fat		Less than	65g	80g
Sat Fat		Less than	20g	25g
Cholesterol		Less than	300mg	300mg
Sodium		Less than	2,400mg	2,400mg
Total Carbohydrate			300g	375g
Dietary Fiber			25g	30g

New Label

Nutrition Facts
8 servings per container
Serving size   2/3 cup (55g)

Amount Per Serving

Calories   230

% **Daily Value***

Total Fat 8g	**10%**
Saturated Fat 1g	**5%**
Trans Fat 0g	
Cholesterol 0mg	**0%**
Sodium 160mg	**7%**
Total Carbohydrate 37g	**13%**
Dietary Fiber 4g	**14%**
Total Sugars 12g	
Includes 10g Added Sugars	**20%**
Protein 3g	

Vitamin D 2mcg	10%
Calcium 260mg	20*
Iron 8mg	45%
Potassium 235 mg	6%

* Percent Daily Values are based on a 2,000 calorie diet. Your daily value may be higher or lower depending on your calorie needs.

Second, the new labels are required to differentiate added sugars from total sugars. Total sugars can be a mix of naturally occurring sugars that come from things like lactose that is naturally present in milk as well as the sugars in any fruit. For example, for a fruit-based yogurt there will be natural sugars from the lactose in the milk as well as from any sugars in the actual fruit. This might be supplemented by any additional added sugars like sucrose or fructose.

With the new food labels, you can determine how much of the sugar in a product like yogurt is from the milk and fruit and how much sugar is added. Added sugars are sugars like sucrose or fructose that are added to a product for additional sweetness. You will have to check the list of ingredients to determine which sugars are added. Keep in mind that ingredient lists are required to be listed in order of the amount contained in a product. So if a sugar of any kind is listed as the first ingredient, then that means that it's the most abundant ingredient in the product. Ideally, for everyday staples, try to find products that do not contain any added sugars. Also, if there are low-calorie sweeteners in the product, it will not show up on the food label itself as added sugar. You will also have to check the ingredient list for any LCS that might be added, as they are required to be listed unless they are present in such small amounts.

How Much Sugar Is Too Much?

You've heard us say that we don't recommend LCS for children. You've heard us talk about which kind of sweetener is best (whole fruit) and what kind is most dangerous (fructose). Now it's time to ask the question: How *much* sugar can children safely consume?

There is no official guideline for how much *total* sugar an adult or child can safely consume—and this is largely because there is no real concern about the sugar that naturally occurs in fruit or dairy. What you really have to focus on is *added* sugar. By this we mean sugar that is added to foods or drinks, such as cane sugar or fruit juice concentrate. Though not everyone would agree that fruit juice is a form of added sugar, we categorize it as such because it is extracted from its whole-food form and contains the sugars from the apple without the fiber. This extracted sugar from fruit is also termed "free" sugars. So we do not consider muffins that are sweetened with a whole blended apple that includes the flesh and skin (fiber) to contain added sugar, but we would consider a glass of apple juice to be a source of added sugars. The US

Department of Agriculture and some other organizations do not, however, count fruit juice as added sugar.

Different organizations have proposed different guidelines for daily added sugar limits. The World Health Organization recommends that adults and children get less than 10 percent of their daily calories from "free" sugars (i.e., added sugars plus sugars from juice), and they state that reducing "free" sugar to 5 percent of daily calories would provide additional health benefits. The United States Department of Agriculture (USDA) has followed suit with a recommendation of less than 10 percent of daily calories for adults and kids, although these guidelines relate to added sugar. If someone consumes 2,000 calories a day, as many adults do, they could consume a maximum of 200 calories of added sugar, or 50 grams. If we stick to the 5 percent guideline, this number would be 100 calories, or 25 grams of added sugar.

It's hard to generalize these guidelines for kids, because energy needs vary by age, and parents usually aren't keeping track of how many calories their kids consume in a day. The guidelines released by the American Heart Association are the only ones specific for children. The AHA recommends zero added sugars for children under two years of age and proposes that children ages two to nineteen consume less than 25 grams per day. This is a useful guide, but not perfect because it groups such a wide age range together. Teens can handle more sugar than toddlers, because they consume more calories.

We believe that parents need a clearer recommendation, one that is tailored to children, so we have created our own set of recommendations based on age. Our Sugarproof guidelines use the 5 percent guideline for "free" and added sugars (as suggested by the WHO) and are based on approximate energy needs of children based on the average weight in each age group. You can use this chart as a general guide to how much added sugar your children should be consuming at maximum. To remind yourself to watch your children's sugar intake, make a copy and stick it on your refrigerator. And to give you a good sense of just how much sugar is in many popular foods, we've provided some information about that, too.

Sugarproof Recommendations for Maximum Daily Added Sugar Intake for Children

Below are our recommendations for daily maximums for added sugar, including sugar from juice. They do not include sugar from whole fruits or vegetables or the naturally occurring lactose in dairy products.

AGE (YEARS)	BOYS	GIRLS
0–2	Zero	Zero
2–3	14g (3½ tsp)	14g (3½ tsp)
3	14g (3½ tsp)	14g (3½ tsp)
4	15g (3¾ tsp)	15g (3¾ tsp)
5	17g (4¼ tsp)	16g (4 tsp)
6	17g (4¼ tsp)	16g (4 tsp)
7	19g (4¾ tsp)	19g (4¾ tsp)
8	20g (5 tsp)	19g (4¾ tsp)
9	20g (5 tsp)	19g (4¾ tsp)
10	20g (5 tsp)	19g (4¾ tsp)
11	23g (5¾ tsp)	21g (5¼ tsp)
12	24g (6 tsp)	22g (5½ tsp)
13	26g (6½ tsp)	23g (5¾ tsp)
14	27g (6¾ tsp)	23g (5¾ tsp)
15	29g (7¼ tsp)	23g (5¾ tsp)
16+ (including adults)	30g (7½ tsp)	24g (6 tsp)

Added Sugars in Common Foods

ITEM	SERVING SIZE	APPROXIMATE ADDED SUGAR
Apple juice box (100%)	6.75 fluid oz.	18–23g
Barbecue sauce	1 tablespoon	6–8g
Blueberry muffin	1 muffin	18–30g
Chewy chocolate chip granola bar	1 bar	7–8g

ITEM	SERVING SIZE	APPROXIMATE ADDED SUGAR
Chocolate chip cookie	1 (26–28g)	8–9g
Chocolate milk	8 fluid oz.	9–11g
Chocolate sandwich cookies	3 cookies	12–14g
Cinnamon raisin bagel	1 bagel	6–7g
Cocoa-flavored cereal (rice or corn based)	1 cup	12–16g
Cola	12-fluid-oz. can	39–41g
Crunchy oat and honey granola bar	1 package	9–11g
Frosted corn flakes cereal	1 cup	12–13g
Frosted toaster pastry	2 pastries	30–39g
Fruit punch	8 fluid oz.	13–14g
Fruit roll snack	1 roll	6–12g
Graham crackers	2 crackers	7–8g
Granola	½ cup	10–12g
Gummy fruit snacks	1 pouch	11–17g
Hamburger bun	1 bun	2–4g
Honey Nut O's cereal	1 cup	10–12g
Hot dog bun	1 bun	3–4g
Instant oatmeal packet, brown sugar and maple	1 packet	12–13g
Ketchup	1 tablespoon	3–4g
Lemon-lime soda	12-fluid-oz. can	37–38g
Maple syrup	1 tablespoon	14g
Oat clusters cereal	1 cup	7–8g
Orange juice box (100%)	6.75 fluid oz.	18–26g
Sports drink	12 fluid oz.	21g
Squeezable yogurt	1 tube	6–7g

ITEM	SERVING SIZE	APPROXIMATE ADDED SUGAR
Strawberry yogurt	6 oz.	11–14g
Sweetened iced tea	12 fluid oz.	17–36g
Sweetened rice cakes	2 cakes	6g
Teriyaki sauce	1 tablespoon	2–3g
Toaster waffle (no syrup)	2 waffles	4–6g
Vanilla yogurt	6 oz.	13–14g
Whole-wheat bread	1 slice	2–3g

Note that we consider 100% juice to be a form of added sugar, as it has been removed from its whole-food form. In addition, some items, such as chocolate milk and yogurt, also contain natural sugar, but here we are providing details on the added sugars.

Sugarproof Recommendations

There are literally hundreds of sugars and sweeteners available to kids today. If you're not sure what kind of sugar to use, just follow these simple guidelines:

- Whenever possible, use whole fruits or unsweetened dried fruits to sweeten foods or beverages. For example, adding a piece of a whole banana or a date to a smoothie is a natural way of sweetening it with a whole food, as opposed to adding table sugar or honey. The same can be done for oatmeal, other cereal, yogurt, or baked goods. See our recipes for ideas.

- White sugar, brown sugar, coconut sugar, molasses, maple syrup, and honey should be used sparingly and reserved for making special treats, using half of what is typically suggested in a recipe.

- Avoid all products made with high-fructose corn syrup, agave, fruit juice concentrate, fruit sugar, or crystalline fructose. These deliver a fructose bomb that children's bodies are not built to handle.

- Avoid juice, even juice that you squeeze at home. They are too high in fructose, and they hit children's bloodstreams too quickly. Fruits are for eating, not drinking.

- Avoid all low-calorie sweeteners.

- Be aware that sugar hides on labels, and manufacturers are constantly finding new ways to label sugar and sweeteners. The easiest way to avoid added sugar is to eat mostly whole foods. If you can't, make it a priority to avoid low-calorie sweeteners and high-fructose corn syrup.

- If you've got any questions about how much added sugar your children can safely consume, consult the chart on page 67.

Next, we'll take a look at the ways all these sugars can affect growing children.

Answers to the Clif Bar Challenge: organic brown rice syrup, organic cane syrup, concentrated apple puree, organic invert sugar syrup, apple juice concentrate, organic glucose syrup, barley malt extract, elderberry juice concentrate. In addition, the high fructose sugars include: concentrated apple puree, apple juice concentrate, blueberry puree, elderberry juice concentrate.

To view the scientific references cited
in this chapter, please visit us online at
sugarproofkids.com/bibliography.

CHAPTER THREE

Hyperactive, Moody, Angry, Sleepy, and Still Hungry: Children on Sugar

Do your children throw tantrums when asked to tidy their room? Or storm around the house for no apparent reason? Or are they unable to sit still—until they are suddenly too fatigued to do much at all? Simply put: Too much sugar can wreak havoc on your child's energy level and mood.

In this chapter, we'll describe why a quick release of sugar into the bloodstream can strap your children onto a roller coaster that causes highs and lows. We'll show you how kids on sugar have a harder time sleeping, which in itself can cause problems with behavior and mood. And we'll talk about why it's harder for kids on sugar to regulate their eating habits—and how easy it is for them to get stuck in the vicious cycle of sugar addiction. Even the youngest of children can become wired to crave more sugar, which in turn has consequences for their appetite, behavior, and mood.

What has been documented in the scientific literature rings true at home: Both of us have observed that our own children are much calmer when they stick to a diet that is lower in sugar and free of sugar substitutes. Parents of the children who participate in our research studies often have the same impressions. They suspect that sugar is making their child aggressive, moody, stressed, or fatigued. But it's not until they see their kids off sugar that they become motivated to commit to a lower-sugar diet for their kids and the whole family.

The Sugar Roller Coaster

I've learned to hate birthday parties. After a cupcake and some ice cream, my kid runs wild and inevitably crashes into someone or something. Then we both go home in a bad mood.

If my middle schooler has a sports drink after school, I brace myself. For a while, he won't be able to sit still. Then he'll flop on the couch and say he's too tired to do homework.

If you're a parent, you've probably seen that when kids have sugar, they experience high levels of activity, followed by a sedentary funk. Science backs up your firsthand experience.

Your child's ride on the sugar roller coaster begins with changes in blood glucose. Glucose, or blood sugar, is the essential source of energy for the body's cells. Our bodies can sense fluctuations in blood glucose levels, and kids can be more sensitive to these changes. When we eat complex carbohydrates, such as steel-cut oatmeal, our bodies break them down into glucose (blood sugar) in a slow, regulated manner. Foods that produce this response are ranked low on the glycemic index, which is a measure of how fast the starches in any particular food are broken down into glucose. In contrast, foods that are high on the glycemic index cause blood sugar levels to rise quickly. High glycemic items include simple carbohydrates that are more easily broken down to glucose (like white rice, corn flakes, pancakes, or cookies) or items that contain a lot of sugar (like candy, a glass of orange juice, or a can of soda). A rapid spike of glucose in the bloodstream will provide a temporary burst of energy, but it won't last for long. After the burst comes a slump, a period of lower energy and mood. And since glucose isn't as well regulated by younger children, they're more likely to have these spikes than adults, and their highs may be higher, and their lows may be lower.

Kim, a mom from New York whom we worked with, noticed that her four-year-old son, Henry, was grumpy first thing in the mornings or after naptime. She would give him a glass of juice, thinking that it would energize him and get him moving more quickly after waking up. However, she noticed that after an initial burst of energy, Henry would go right back to being tired and cranky again, often ending up in a worse mood than before his nap. She noticed that the more juice she gave him, the harder the crash.

Henry's body was receiving too much sugar all at once, sending it into overdrive. In response to a high sugar load, the body overcompensates with a big surge of insulin, the hormone that is needed to take the glucose out of the blood and into cells for use as fuel. If too much insulin is dispatched to the scene, the body overreacts. The sudden rise in blood sugar will be shortly followed with an extreme drop, and as blood sugar drops, so does energy level and often mood. This is the classic sugar crash. Henry was essentially getting on board the sugar roller coaster first thing each morning, and sometimes after his nap as well.

Different Breakfasts = Different Behaviors

Take dozens of teenagers, give them different things to eat or drink, and then see if they succumb to the sugar roller coaster. This was the premise of an ingenious study led by a colleague at USC, Dr. Donna Spruijt-Metz, and we were lucky to help out. The research team asked eighty-seven overweight teens if they would like to volunteer for a study. They were given two separate breakfasts on two separate days. The first consisted of a Pop Tart, a Tampico orange juice drink, and a reduced-fat string cheese. This was designed to be high in sugar and low in fiber. The second breakfast was designed to have the same number of calories but was low in sugar and high in fiber: a whole-wheat bagel with margarine and a glass of water with a fiber supplement. After eating each meal, the teens went to a room that was stocked with treadmills, mini-trampolines, motion-based video games, jump ropes, free weights, a TV, art supplies, music devices, and more. Each teen wore an accelerometer, a device that measures activity levels, and we monitored the volunteers periodically for blood sugar levels.

After the high-sugar meal, the teens were all over the place. First they tended to select active options like walking on the treadmill, then they switched to something sedentary, like sitting and watching a movie. Then they jumped up and became active again. But after the meal that was low in sugar and high in fiber, the teens' activity levels were much more stable. They tended to pick one type of activity and stick to it. And as we suspected, the fluctuations in activity levels after the high-sugar meal were mirrored with similar fluctuations in blood sugar levels. During the first ninety minutes after eating, higher than average blood sugar levels were linked to higher activity.

Similar results have been observed in younger children, too. It might even be more pronounced. In one study, preschool children were given orange juice sweetened with sucrose. Forty to fifty-five minutes later, they were less able to sit still in class, had more inappropriate behavior, and had more difficulty concentrating. Overall, the research delivers a simple and practical message. Give kids a lower-sugar diet, and they will experience steadier energy levels and most likely a sharper focus.

Sugar and Excitability: Is It All in Your Mind?

You might have heard that the link between sugar and activity levels is all in your mind, and that your kids seem more hyper after sugar simply because you expect them to be. Not so. This myth is based on outdated information, but it's still going strong—we hear it from parents on a regular basis—so we'll take a moment to bust it.

Some of this stems from an old study that was published in the *Journal of the American Medical Association*. This 1995 paper looked at twenty-three previous studies that examined the effects of sugar consumption on children's behavior and energy levels, and it concluded that sugar had no clear effects. But we've learned a lot since 1995. The data that was available had several limitations. The main problem with this analysis was that all of the studies that were reviewed compared the effects of sugar to the effects of a low-calorie sweetener as a control. In all of these studies, an LCS was used as the placebo comparison group with the assumption that they would have no effect of their own. If kids' behavior is the same after consuming both sugar and LCS, the researchers reasoned, the sugar must not have an effect on behavior at all. Now we know better. Low-calorie sweeteners mimic sugar so well that children's brains and bodies often can't tell the difference. Aspartame, for example, causes an increase in both gross and fine motor movement. Why? Low-calorie sweeteners activate the same receptors, both in the brain and throughout the body, that real sugars do. These receptors can trigger a cascade of hormone release that impacts behavior. The second major problem with the analysis is that a number of the kids who were studied had been diagnosed with attention deficit/hyperactivity disorder (ADHD), aggressive behaviors, or psychiatric problems. One study even included children with Prader–Willi syndrome, a rare genetic disorder that can affect appetite, metabolism, development, and behavior. It would be hard to draw any firm conclusions from such diverse groups of children.

Finally, the 1995 analysis was based on studies that were not consistent when it came to how kids actually consumed the sugar. In some studies, the kids were fed sugar after an overnight fast; some were given it with breakfast; and some mixed it into a glass of orange juice that already contained natural sugar of its own. One study provided children with a high-sugar diet over a period of three weeks and then brought the kids in for general observation instead of feeding them sugar and performing an immediate observation, the way the other studies did. It's hard to get good comparative data when the methodologies vary so widely. If someone tells you that the sugar-behavior connection is all in your mind, remember: You can trust your own observations, and you know when your child is amped up from too much sugar.

The Unpredictable Effects of Sugar

Have you ever noticed that sometimes your children become agitated after sugar, and sometimes they don't? Or maybe you have two children who respond differently to the exact same sugary food or drink. That's often because a child's response to sugar depends on what is consumed along with the sugar. If you've ever eaten a piece of cake as a snack in the middle of the afternoon, you've probably noticed a stronger sugar rush than when you have the same cake after a meal. Sugar has a high glycemic index, but if it is combined with fat or protein, it is digested more slowly and does not raise blood sugar as quickly.

And sometimes children respond in different ways to sugar for no apparent reason. The same child may not process a set amount of sugar in the same way on two different days. Even in standardized clinical tests performed in a hospital setting for diabetes or prediabetes, children who have fasted overnight and then consumed a standard dose of sugar can have different blood glucose responses on two different days. This variation is not uncommon and is one of the reasons that testing children for diabetes—and conducting real-life experiments about sugar consumption—is so difficult. Children may test positive on one day and negative on another. A thorough diagnosis requires a positive test on two separate occasions. Scientists aren't sure why the results can be so variable, but factors such as stress, sleep, or lingering effects from the previous day's meal may play a role.

The individual day-to-day variations in how sugar is processed may also be more pronounced in kids because they are still developing the ability to regulate blood glucose, particularly after consuming large amounts of sugar. You are probably familiar with how your children's behavior changes from day to day, or even minute to minute. The same is true for how they respond to sugar; their responses can be different on different days. And often one sibling can be more sensitive to sugar than the other. In the second part of this book, we'll offer you strategies and plans for reducing the sugar in your children's diet. We encourage you to play the role of scientist in your own home by collecting your own data on how everyone responds to changes in reducing sugar.

Sugar and ADHD

"I'm so confused. Does sugar cause ADHD, or not?"

We frequently hear questions like this one from parents of children who have been diagnosed with attention deficit/hyperactivity disorder (ADHD). In the hopes of helping their kids, these parents have consulted websites, books, friends, and physicians. In short, they've been told two things:

1. Sugar causes ADHD.

2. Sugar does not cause ADHD.

We don't blame these parents for feeling exasperated. And there are plenty of parents who wonder how to get at the truth of sugar's role in ADHD. Attention deficit/hyperactivity disorder affects 9 percent of children in the United States, according to a report from the Centers for Disease Control and Prevention, and the number of children diagnosed has increased steadily over the past decades.

At this point, there is no clear evidence that a high-sugar diet causes ADHD in kids. But it's also premature to completely rule out sugar as a factor in kids' impulsiveness, lack of focus, or hyperactivity. That's because some preliminary research does suggest that a poor overall diet is linked to ADHD and that a balanced diet can reduce a child's risk of developing it. A study that looked at the diets of almost two thousand Australian kids is especially interesting. Australia is heavily influenced by Asian and Pacific Rim countries as well as Western cultures, so researchers there are able to look at children who have a wide variety of diets and traditions. The children who ate a more Western-style diet—which is high in fat, sugar, and salt and low in omega-3 fatty acids, fiber, and folate—were more likely to have ADHD than kids who followed a more traditional Asian or Pacific Rim diet. A smaller study conducted in Spain found similar results, showing that habits like skipping breakfast, eating at fast-food restaurants, and consuming sugar, candy, cola beverages, and noncola soft drinks were associated with a diagnosis of ADHD.

Is there enough evidence for scientists to pronounce a clear link between sugar and ADHD? No. But is there a reason for parents to reduce the sugar intake of kids with ADHD? Of course. We know that sugar and LCS can increase kids' tendency to be hyperactive, so it is possible that sugars/LCS can exacerbate ADHD. Reducing sugar might not be a proven treatment for ADHD, but it certainly can't hurt to try. Doctors often suggest an elimination diet to see whether food allergies or sensitivities, particularly to food dyes or preservatives, are making symptoms worse. We think it's also worth cutting out added sugars for a while, just to see what happens. Families struggling with ADHD in their children and who want to reduce sugar might appreciate the structure offered by either our 7-Day Challenge or the 28-Day Challenge. Of course, you should follow your doctor's advice about treatments for ADHD.

Mad and Sad: How Sugar Affects Mood, Temperament, and Stress Levels

Take a moment to ponder this important question: Do you know what your children are like *without* sugar? Most parents don't realize how daily sugar consumption shapes their kids' mood and disposition. You may have become so used to how your children act on sugar that you have accepted it as part of who they are. Take Valentina, who described her four-year-old daughter Olivia as "generally explosive," a "bad tantrum-thrower," and "a child who likes to soothe herself with food." As she learned about sugar and examined her child's diet, Valentina uncovered a pattern. "I'm practically drip-feeding Olivia sugar throughout the day," she told us with surprise. The major culprits were the waffles with syrup at breakfast, yogurt with chocolate chips for a mid-morning snack, and a yogurt drink (with added sugar) in a small bottle for afternoon snack.

Valentina and her family began our 7-Day Challenge—and at first, Olivia was angry when her favorite snacks were replaced with lower-sugar alternatives. It seemed as if her bad mood wasn't getting any better. But by the end of the week, Olivia began to go along with the new plan. It helped that her family was making the same changes along with her. And better still, Olivia began to calm down. Valentina had never suspected that some of her daughter's behavior had been driven by sugar.

Maybe you've already noticed your children are crankier or more oppositional when they have sugar. But the changes to a child's overall disposition can be even more extensive than many parents suspect, primarily because of the way sugars signal different parts of the brain. Sugar affects multiple parts of the brain and has effects on cognitive skills, self-control, memory, and mood and produces a feeling of craving more. TED-Ed created a useful animated video called *How Sugar Affects the Brain* that you can find on their website. Sugar's messages to the brain start almost immediately after the taste receptors in your mouth register something sweet. It's like an online transaction. Once you click on "send" or "buy now," you can't reverse the process. Even if you swirled around a big mouthful of soda and spat it out, the sugar molecules will have already acted on the taste receptors and signaled the brain. The same goes for LCS, because they trigger the same receptors. Once these receptors are activated, they send a signal to the brain stem and then to the cerebral cortex where the sweet taste is registered. Then a signal is sent to the reward system, which senses pleasure and triggers a response to want more. Sugar consumption also causes an increase in dopamine levels, which have a similar effect on the reward system.

The idea that sugar affects mood may seem like a logical conclusion, but the parents we work with are still surprised at the positive results they see when their kids cut down on sugar. Emma, for example, was eight years old and often grumpy. She stomped around the house in the mornings and rattled her family with her bad moods. Emma's mother, Gina, was already worried about what Emma would be like as a teenager. However, by day five of our 7-Day Challenge, Emma was less moody. Emma's personality seemed more even. Gina said with relief, "It was really nice to see."

Paige and Shelby, ages twelve and fourteen, were two sisters who had very different interests and talents, but they had developed something striking in common: They were both constantly irritable. ("Irritability" is the rather genteel term psychologists use for "easily angered, stressed, and frustrated.") Their parents had become frustrated with both girls' moods and inability to cope with minor problems. The family followed a healthy-sounding diet that they believed was low in sugar. However, a closer look revealed that coconut water and sweets made with stevia and other sweeteners were daily staples. Once the girls backed off these high doses of sugar and low-calorie sweeteners, their moods stabilized dramatically.

My colleagues at the University of Southern California performed an experiment designed to understand the sugar–mood connection. Children between the ages of nine and thirteen were given mobile devices, which would beep every now and then with these questions:

How STRESSED were you feeling just before the beep went off?

How MAD were you feeling just before the beep went off?

How NERVOUS OR ANXIOUS were you feeling just before the beep went off?

How SAD were you feeling just before the beep went off?

The team examined the associations between the kids' answers and what they were eating. The children who ate a lot of added sugar were much more stressed, angry, anxious, and sad; kids who ate less sugar were more stable. Moreover, the sugared-up kids had more extreme emotional reactions, experiencing both higher highs and lower lows in a fashion that must have exhausted both them and their parents.

High sugar consumption contributes to other aspects of kids' moods and mental health, including depression. Studies have found connections between national levels of sugar consumption and national prevalence of disorders in anxiety, mood, impulse control, and substance abuse and even schizophrenia. And a large study tracked the diets in eight thousand adults over twenty-two years. Men who consumed more than 67 grams of sugar per day were 23 percent more likely to have a diagnosis of depression after five years than men who consumed less than 40 grams of sugar per day. These studies aren't linked to children specifically, but they suggest that all of us should be concerned about how sugar can affect our mood and mental health.

The one sugar habit that has the biggest impact on mental well-being is regular consumption of sweetened beverages. A large meta-analysis of studies around the globe found that drinking tea and coffee was generally protective for depression, whereas regular consumption of sugary beverages was related to a 36 percent higher risk. Although this study was not specific to children, the findings are still relevant to the dangers of sugar for kids. The results were not affected by age of the subjects, gender, or country where the study was conducted. Another study conducted with 5,498 tenth graders in Norway found that regular consumption of sugar-sweetened beverages was linked not only to hyperactivity and behavior problems but also to mental distress and mental difficulties.

Why is sugar linked to mental distress in teens? Adolescence is a critical period for development of the hypothalamic pituitary adrenal (HPA) axis, a part of the brain involved with how our bodies coordinate response to stress. Studies in animals show that a higher consumption of sugars, fructose in particular, during this critical period can magnify stress responses. For example, rats that are given a high-fructose diet for ten weeks show indications of anxiety-related behavior, depression, and elevated stress hormones. (Yes, rats in cages do get stressed, and scientists use various measures, such as how much they socialize, or how long they explore novel objects that are introduced, or how they respond to bright light, to gauge it.) Fructose acted by turning on certain genes in the HPA axis that made them more likely to be stressed. Moreover, this response was unique to adolescent rats; adult mice were not affected by the same fructose exposure. The fructose specifically affected the developing brains of the adolescent rats.

Studies suggest clear links between sugars in the diet and your child's mood and mental well-being. We think it's time to revise the old adage "you are what you eat." We should also tell our kids, "you *feel* how you eat."

Forget about Sweet Dreams: Sleepless on Sugar

Some of my (Michael's) most memorable experiences as a parent have been accompanying my kids on school camping trips, trekking in Anza Borrego and hiking into slot canyons in Utah. My one issue with these trips? Every night, on every trip, after the evening campfire and before bed, the teachers handed out brownies to the kids. The kids worked hard, and I certainly wouldn't want to deny them a treat on a special occasion like this one. The problem is the timing: They gave the kids brownies right before they went off to their tents for the night. If you have ever been on a camping trip with kids, you know that they tend to have a hard time settling down in tents. It's hard enough without a jolt of chocolate and sugar. You can imagine the results: The boys waged war on neighboring tents. They played loud games with their flash-lights. They screamed that they saw wild animals. After those brownies, no one got a decent night's sleep.

Losing a night or two of sleep on a camping trip isn't a big deal, just as having brownies now and then isn't a big deal. But over time, sleep loss can become a big problem. When kids don't get enough sleep, they're more likely to develop obesity and related diseases like diabetes and cardiovascular disease. Babies who don't sleep at least twelve hours a day have a greater risk of being overweight by three years of age, and some research connects teen sleep deprivation with depression.

Plenty of kids have dessert before bed almost every night, which can interrupt their sleep. In some families, sweet beverages are served because they're thought to have relaxing effects. Think of hot chocolate before bed or the juice bottles or sippy cups that parents give infants or toddlers to relax them before they settle down for the night. I (Emily) lived for a while in Italy, where having chamomile tea is a nightly ritual for many families, and most Italians enjoy theirs sweetened. Sugary, granulated chamomile tea powders are even sold specifically for dissolving in warm water for baby bottles, and this drink is believed to have soothing effects for infants. In actuality, these sweet nighttime beverages could be making their kids' sleep worse (not to mention that they contribute to tooth decay).

Too much sugar right before bedtime will cause an energy spike, delaying the time for settling down. It can also interfere with sleep patterns by reducing melatonin secretion and disturbing the normal circadian rhythm. This sets up a vicious cycle. Less sleep at night leads to being more tired the next day and being more tired tends to lead to cravings for more sugar, which in turn leads to less sleep. Our bodies intuitively seek out additional energy from food to keep us going when we are tired, and often we turn to something sweet because it might give us a quicker burst of energy. Research shows that teens who are already short on sleep will increase their energy intake, especially from snacking on foods high in sugar. And any parent will tell you that when nighttime sleep is less restful and restorative, it's tough for everyone. It's harder to maintain an even temper. Lack of sleep directly relates to performance during the day, whether it's falling asleep in class or underperforming on the sports team.

It's even possible that high amounts of sugar can be detrimental to sleep *no matter what time of the day they are consumed.* One large study of nearly six thousand kids ages nine through eleven showed that kids with lower levels of soft drink consumption were more likely to sleep the recommended nine to eleven hours per night and on average got twelve more minutes of sleep. Twelve minutes of sleep might not sound like much, but remember that's an average spread out over thousands of children, so for some children, sleep loss might be thirty minutes or more. We don't know for sure if this reduced sleep is due to the sugar or the caffeine that tends to also be high in many carbonated soft drinks. Either way, avoiding soft drinks, no matter what the caffeine level, is a wise idea for both adults and kids.

The Sleep-Stealing, Heart-Thumping Effects of Energy Drinks

You've seen the comically garish labels and intense brand names: Monster. Rockstar. Amp. Bang. These marketing techniques practically sing out to teens, who love their energy drinks. They're used by an estimated 30 percent of adolescents and 50 percent of young adults. Energy drinks generally contain high amounts of caffeine along with sugar (or an LCS) and ingredients considered dietary supplements, such as taurine and ginseng. Some teens consciously use these drinks to boost and maintain their energy. They drink them while studying for long hours, participating in a marathon video gaming session, or getting through the early morning during a summer job. Some teens buy energy drinks just because they like them and they seem cool.

A can of soda might contain 50 milligrams of caffeine. A cup of coffee contains about 100 milligrams. But a typical energy drink might contain anywhere from 70 to 200 milligrams of caffeine.

For most adults, drinking the equivalent of a few cups of coffee is perfectly safe. But teens are still growing, and their bodies are different. The American Academy of Pediatrics recommends no more than 100 milligrams of caffeine per day for teens. This limit could easily be exceeded with one energy drink alone.

The double whammy of the caffeine plus the high content of sugar means that energy drinks are especially addictive. The more kids drink them, the more they want them, and the more withdrawal they experience when they don't get their fix. These brain bombs lead to all the usual problems that too much sugar can bring, including poor sleep. Plus, teens will feel the usual aftereffects of high doses of caffeine and other stimulants. Even the brightest and most focused of teens might need you to remind them that energy drinks contain caffeine and that both caffeine and sugar can disrupt their sleep. They might need you to spell out some of the commonly reported side effects, including headaches, heart palpitations, feeling jittery, and abdominal pain. For all of these reasons, you can tell your teen, the American Academy of Pediatrics does not recommend energy drinks at all for children or teenagers, and neither do we.

What about Sports Drinks?

In contrast to energy drinks, sports drinks often contain electrolytes (such as sodium or potassium) and carbohydrates in the form of sucrose, glucose, or fructose. They're designed to help high-performance athletes recover more quickly, especially during hot weather or high-intensity workouts or games. The electrolytes help the body absorb fluids more quickly than drinking regular water and help prevent dehydration. The original sports drink was developed by the College of Medicine at the University of Florida to enhance recovery and replenishment for the champion Gators football team; hence the name Gatorade.

These drinks have gone mainstream and multiplied in the market today. But the vast majority of teens who drink them simply don't need the added sugars, and they definitely don't need the fructose. Sure, some high school athletes begin their seasons in the high heat of summer with rigorous training workouts and games in which replenishment of electrolytes is especially important. For these teens, an occasional sports drink might make sense. But teens who engage in shorter, less intense workouts, or who are simply hanging out with friends, do not need them. Nor do they need the lower- or no-calorie versions of these drinks. While most don't carry the caffeine load of an energy drink, they still count as a sweet beverage for kids who simply don't need the extra sugar/sweetener burden.

I'm Still Hungry! Sugar and Overeating

Have you ever described your child as a "bottomless pit"? Sometimes a child's big appetite can be related to a growth spurt or a strenuous day of physical activity. But sometimes there may be days of what seems like nonstop hunger and eating intertwined with irritable outbursts. If this pattern seems familiar, stop and take a moment the next time it happens. Consider what your child has had to eat or drink that day. It could be that sugar has increased your child's appetite or, worse yet, has provoked a type of emergency hunger that makes your child feel an urgent, overwhelming need to eat.

This panicky hunger is brought to you by insulin, the hormone that is released by the pancreas. When you eat, your blood sugar rises, and your pancreas sends insulin into your blood. There, insulin clears glucose from the blood and sends it into the cells that need it for energy. If insulin is doing its job effectively, your blood sugar levels will fall slowly. But if you eat something that's high in sugar or other carbohydrates, your blood sugar can rise quickly and extra insulin can be dispatched in response, causing your blood sugar to fall *too* quickly. This can cause a state of hypoglycemia (low blood sugar). The body senses depleting energy levels and goes into panic mode. You feel shaky and irritable. You feel an urge to eat more food, quickly, to regain your equilibrium. In other words, you're *hangry*—even if you've just eaten, thanks to the way your body responds to sugar or simple carbohydrates. The same goes for kids, except that they are less likely to understand why they feel so bad and so hungry. Sweet drinks or foods high in sugar or other simple carbohydrates that rapidly break down to sugar lead to the biggest up-and-down swings of blood glucose levels. Avoiding sweet drinks and switching to foods that are high in fiber, protein, and healthy fats will help kids feel full for longer periods and help break this cycle.

Certain kinds of sugar can disrupt the parts of the brain responsible for sensing that calories have been consumed, which can make your kids feel hungry even after they've just eaten. One of my colleagues at USC, Dr. Katie Page, gave healthy adults either fructose or glucose. Then she put them in an MRI machine and measured the activity in different parts of their brains. The two different sugars led to very different patterns of activity in the regions of the brain that are related to appetite and reward. The volunteers who'd taken the glucose showed patterns related to feelings of fullness and satiety—which is what you'd expect after a snack. But the brains of the people who'd taken the fructose were showing entirely the opposite. The hypothalamus, a key area for regulating food intake and energy balance, did not even register the fructose as caloric intake.

Nor did the striatum, another area of the brain that helps us sense when we're full. It was as if the brain failed to understand that the calories from the fructose had been consumed. These volunteers did not feel full or satiated. They were still hungry. Rat studies have shown similar results. When glucose is injected directly into their brains, they slow down their feeding. When fructose is injected, the rats keep on eating.

While fructose appears to cause overeating, it's not the only sweet substance that keeps your child feeling hungry even after eating. Low-calorie sweeteners (LCS) can also create false impressions in the brain about food intake. Since LCS do not provide any calories, they don't deliver the feeling of fullness that the body expects when eating or drinking. LCS leave you with an unfulfilled desire for calories, which can cause compensatory overeating during other parts of the day. That explains why another study of more than seven thousand kids found that children who drink LCS beverages end up consuming 200 more calories throughout the day than children who drink water. Kids who drank both sugary beverages and LCS beverages had it even worse. They consumed an additional 450 calories throughout the day, above and beyond the extra calories from the soda.

Worse, consuming LCS on a regular basis can have a cumulative effect. With time, it can erode our overall ability to sense caloric intake, meaning that the brain no longer associates eating or drinking *anything* sweet with actually receiving calories. A Yale University study found that the more artificial sweeteners that people consume in their regular diet, the less their brains respond when they are given actual sugar that does contain calories. Bottom line: Fructose and LCS confuse children's bodies, making it harder for them to feel full, even after eating.

No Joke: The Vicious Cycle of Craving More

I (Emily) was at a birthday party the other day. I was standing near the dessert table, where cakes, cupcakes, and doughnut holes were laid out in sumptuous display. A father watched as his daughter took some of each. At first he moved to stop the child, but she protested. The dad put his hands in the air in surrender, then shrugged as if to say, *She's a kid at a party. What can a parent do?* Then he said to the other adults with a sigh, "My kid's such a sugar addict."

He was joking. But sugar actually *is* just like a drug, especially in the way it works on the brain—and especially the way it works on kids' brains. The effects of sugar on the body and the brain are strikingly similar to those of other addictive substances. Do you recognize any of these symptoms in your children?

- Tendency to overconsume sugar (bingeing)
- Headaches and moodiness if they try to give up sugar (withdrawal symptoms)
- Craving more sugar
- Tolerance to the effects of sugar
- Difficulty cutting back on sugar

The symptoms are all included in the clinical criteria for addiction. When we eat or drink sugar or something sweet, the flavor has strong and stimulating effects on the reward center of the brain. This reward center is responsible for synthesizing and releasing dopamine, the "feel good" neurotransmitter. The reward center also produces and releases natural opioids. Although these body-generated opioids are safe—and much different than illegal or medically prescribed opiates—they generate strong feelings of pleasure and reward. Together, dopamine and these natural opioids give the body strong feelings of well-being. So it comes as no surprise that drinking or eating sugar gives you this same feeling, and that experience can develop into a craving to generate it again and again. Sugar generates chemical signals in your brain that make you feel good, which translates in behavioral terms to wanting more. This process is magnified in children because they already have a built-in stronger preference for sweetness.

In our studies, when we first ask kids to cut back on sugar, a frequent answer is that "something will be missing." This intangible "something" is the good feeling that makes sugar so desirable—and creates a habit that is difficult to break. Another factor that makes sugar consumption difficult to shake is that there is a direct link between the amount of sugar consumed and the number of dopamine receptors that are activated in the brain. What this means is that the brain requires more and more sugar to produce the same level of good feelings. Just like with addictive drugs, over time it takes larger doses to get that high, or sense of reward in the brain. In fact, the drive to consume sugar can become so powerful that some young people in our studies have said that they literally can't imagine going without it.

Once sugar addiction sets in, withdrawal symptoms may become apparent in much the same way as they would with an addiction to alcohol or hard drugs. In a classic animal study, researchers showed that lab rats prefer sugar and artificial sweeteners over cocaine. One study looked at the differences in how rats responded to Oreo cookies in particular versus cocaine or morphine. They found that the Oreo cookies had a stronger effect on activating a certain part of the brain that is connected to addiction and reward, the *nucleus accumbens*. Obviously, we cannot perform these kinds of studies in kids (or adults), and therefore the jury is still out on the strength of sugar addiction relative to other addictive drugs in humans. But the animal evidence is shocking.

There are parents who notice some of the signs of sugar addiction in their kids. Even if they don't know the research, they've noticed the bingeing, the craving, the moodiness. In response, they move their children onto drinks and snacks sweetened with LCS. Why not, they think? Low-calorie sweeteners might be bad, but they're not *as* bad, and at least they're helping kids kick the sugar habit, right? When these families come into our clinic, one of the first things we do is break the bad news about LCS. Aside from the chemical risks that are simply not yet fully understood, LCS trick the brain into thinking they're real sugars, which contributes to the cycle of craving sweetness and overeating. Artificial sweeteners like sucralose have addictive properties that are similar to sugar's, and they can activate some of the same reward pathways of the brain that are so problematic. All LCS activate sweet taste receptors in the mouth and throughout the body. The activation of these sweet taste receptors initiates a cascade of events that will happen whether or not they are triggered by real sugar, fake sugar, or a naturally occurring low-calorie sweetener. In one study, a group of college students drank either Sprite Zero (sweetened with aspartame), regular Sprite, or plain sparkling water. Then they were offered a choice of M&M's, a bottle of spring water, or a pack of Trident sugar-free gum. The students who had the Sprite Zero with aspartame were nearly three times more likely to choose the M&M's than the students who were given either of the other two beverages. In this case, the LCS didn't just mimic sugar's ability to cause cravings. It was *more powerful*.

As parents, we have to do the hard work of breaking not just the sugar-addiction cycle but the sweet-taste addiction cycle as well.

Tiny Sugar Addicts

Sugar addiction can begin in utero. The central reward system of the brain begins to develop as early as twelve weeks of gestation, and by twenty weeks, receptors for dopamine and opioids can be detected. Since glucose can cross the placenta, any excess sugar a mom consumes during pregnancy could affect the developing brain by triggering these newly formed receptors. In theory, the brain can become hardwired to have a stronger desire for more sugar. In other words, the innate preference for sweetness that babies are born with could become stronger based on the sugars that moms eat even before birth. While we don't yet have evidence from studies in humans, several animal studies support this idea and also show that LCS have a similar effect. Based on what we know, we advise moderation of sugar and avoidance of LCS intake during pregnancy.

Your Kids Need Your Support

The addictive power of sugar and LCS can be strong enough to get in the way of healthy choices, even in the face of frightening health consequences. That's why kids usually can't rightsize their sugar intake on their own; they need you to help. Earlier in the book, we introduced you to Marco, a high school athlete who was diagnosed with fatty liver disease, a serious disorder that can eventually result in the need for a liver transplant. Marco was part of a twelve-week program we'd designed. He met with a dietician four times, was provided with nutritional information and strategies focused on cutting back on sugar, and he received a delivery of bottled water to his home every week. But despite this help, he had many challenges. For one, he was on the football team and felt that as an athlete, he needed calories and could eat and drink whatever he wanted. Also, his friends on the team bonded around eating and drinking. As he said, it was "more important to fit in and drink sodas with friends than to avoid them as a way to improve my liver." Marco will tell you that he understands that both his liver and his overall health will get better if he kicks his habit. Then he'll admit that he continues to drink sodas and energy drinks anyway, especially when his family orders fast-food meals like tacos or hamburgers. The combination of carbohydrates (including sugar) and fat produce an even stronger feeling of pleasure and sense of reward together than either of them on their own. Marco craves soda with his fast-food meals because the combination of fat and carbohydrate is a powerful activator of the reward response and sets up an expectation in the brain that feeds the addiction. When we ask Marco why he drinks so many energy drinks and sodas, he says, "They just taste good," and from the light in his eyes it's clear how much reward Marco gets from sugar.

Marco's situation tells a powerful story of the realities of sugar addiction. Although Marco was not able to reduce sugar during our twelve-week study, the majority of kids do make significant improvements, and in Chapter 5 we will introduce you to a couple of other kids who were able to successfully reduce sugar and improve their health. Marco didn't have the support of either friends or family as he tried to kick the sugar habit, and that made things much, much harder for him. Even teens need help from their parents as they try to change the way they approach food.

At any level of sugar intake, when sugar is eliminated or even grad-ually reduced, you will likely notice physiological signs of withdrawal such as headaches, anxiety, and anger. Older kids or teens may be able to communicate with you about what they are feeling when cutting back sugar, but young children are not as likely to be able to explain what is going on in their body and may get angry or have a tantrum instead. Recognizing these withdrawal effects will become important as you reduce sugar. Don't worry, because we'll show you plenty of tested ways to inspire your kids and create the supportive environment they need to reset their sugar preferences for better health.

To view the scientific references cited in this chapter, please visit us online at sugarproofkids.com/bibliography.

CHAPTER FOUR

Smarter without Sugar: Sugar's Effects on Learning, Memory, and the Growing Brain

If you could look at the brains of healthy adults who typically drink one or two sodas per day and compare them to the brains of people who drink less than one per day, you would see something astonishing. The brains of the group drinking sugary beverages would be smaller. To put it bluntly, new research shows that too much sugar shrinks your brain.

It's only recently that we have begun to understand the effects of sugar on the brain—on its size, volume, architecture, and ability to function. And it's only *very* recently that new research is shining a light onto the incredibly damaging effects that sugar can have on the growing brains of children and teens.

Too much sugar impairs children's abilities to excel at their tasks, whether it's building a tower of blocks at age two, writing an essay for a college application at age seventeen, or taking standardized tests in the classroom at any age. Kids who consume high amounts of sugar and sweeteners simply aren't as sharp as they could be. They have trouble concentrating. It's harder for them to remember to bring their notebooks home from school, or to recall things like the dates of the Vietnam War for a history test.

The effects of too much sugar don't stop with reduced academic achievement. Kids who consume too much sugar are less able to control their impulses, which can have serious consequences, especially for teenagers. Teens with a sugar habit tend to make poor decisions—and because this age group is already prone to taking risks, those poor decisions can have lasting consequences. Furthermore, an early sugar habit can reshape the brain permanently and put kids at risk for disorders later in life, including early cognitive decline and future risk of Alzheimer's disease.

This chapter will show you the research—my own as well as some of my colleagues, and other experts—that links too much sugar and sweeteners to problems ranging from mental focus to one of the most feared neurodegenerative disorders of our time. But it's not all bad news. When you know that sugar could be the reason a child is exhibiting difficult behavior or not performing up to his or her ability, you have the power to change the outcome.

Is Your Child Struggling in School?

A New Jersey–based mom named Elizabeth and her husband received an e-mail from their daughter's eighth grade science teacher that said, "I just wanted to touch base because I am a little concerned about Grace. The other day she was falling asleep in science class. This is not the first time that I noticed this happening."

The message was a huge surprise to Grace's parents. Science was second period, which started at 9:00 a.m. How could Grace, who was a bright, straight-A student, be so tired by then? Elizabeth and her husband felt that Grace's 9:30 p.m. bedtime was reasonable for a fourteen-year-old, but they figured she must not be getting enough sleep. So they told her that she needed to go to bed even earlier and that there would be a new rule of no phone use after 7:00 p.m. to reduce blue light exposure. Despite these efforts, Grace still struggled to stay awake mid-morning. Something just wasn't right, and her parents and her teacher couldn't seem to figure it out.

Flash-forward to later that year, when Elizabeth and her family participated in our 7-Day No-Added-Sugar Challenge. As part of this, Grace changed her breakfast routine. She would usually have Honey Nut Cheerios (12 grams or 3 teaspoons added sugars per cup) with whole milk and a glass of a 100 percent juice blend of peach, mango, and orange (24 grams or 6 teaspoons of added sugars per cup). Plus, she would take her daily gummy multivitamin and a calcium plus vitamin D chew (3 grams or ¾ teaspoon). That's almost 40 grams or 10 teaspoons of added sugars at breakfast alone, which is almost twice her daily maximum recommendation of 23 grams (5¾ teaspoons). That's not even including the second helping of cereal Grace would regularly serve herself because she still felt hungry after the first bowl.

During the 7-Day Challenge with zero added sugars, Grace instead had unsweetened oatmeal with raspberries, almond meal, and pecans for breakfast, and she skipped the juice and sugar-sweetened vitamins. Suddenly, Grace could easily stay awake in second period. That's when it all started to click: Grace was eating a sugar bomb of a breakfast at 7:30 a.m., and by 9:00 a.m., she was crashing. It was her morning food choices, not her bedtime routine, that was causing her drowsiness.

Grace's twelve-year-old sister, Tiffany, saw immediate benefits from a change in her breakfast as well. Her preferred breakfast on the 7-Day Challenge was scrambled eggs with cheddar cheese and toast, something she could even make herself. Tiffany, who has ADHD, commented to her mom that on the days when she eats eggs for breakfast, she is better able to concentrate in class, and that she should be sure to have them on days when she has tests.

Elizabeth feels fortunate that they were able to put two and two together and that her daughters are doing well with their new breakfast routine. In addition to causing spikes and dips in energy levels, high amounts of sugar at breakfast disrupt a child's focus, concentration, and memory. In contrast, breakfasts without added sugars that are high in protein and fiber help stabilize blood sugar levels throughout the morning. We will have much more to say in later chapters that provide strategies for a Sugarproof breakfast.

Focus and Concentration

It might come as a surprise, given everything we've just said about sugar, but the brain does need sugar to function. In fact, the brain's main fuel is the basic sugar glucose. But this doesn't mean you need to eat straight sugar to give your brain the glucose it needs. In an ideal situation, the body gets this glucose from a variety of foods. The best source of glucose is that released from the slow, steady breakdown of complex carbohydrates, including whole grains, legumes, fruits, and vegetables. Glucose circulates in your blood and is what we know as blood sugar. It crosses the blood–brain barrier, and once in the brain, it fuels the neurons (brain cells) and helps them transmit and receive information. If you are healthy, your body does a good job of keeping your blood glucose levels within a certain range that keeps your brain functioning in a healthy zone. This is largely thanks to hormones like insulin that regulate your blood sugar.

Even still, your body and your brain are very sensitive to fluctuations in blood glucose. When you eat complex carbohydrates, your body breaks them down into glucose in a slow, regular manner. This helps keep your blood sugar levels steady. But when you eat or drink something with simple carbohydrates that are more easily broken down to glucose (like white rice, corn flakes, pancakes, or cookies) or that contain a lot of plain sugar (like a glass of orange juice or a can of soda), your blood sugar spikes. At first, this is likely to boost your brain function. Research shows that right after you drink a sugary beverage, you are better able to complete tasks that involve processing information, resolving conflict, and recalling words. But because your body has received too much sugar all at once, it goes into overdrive and like we described in Chapter 3, you likely board the sugar roller coaster. In response to the sugar load, it overcompensates with a big surge of insulin. This flood of insulin can cause an extreme drop in your blood sugar. You already know that as your blood sugar drops, so do your energy levels. But your mental performance can drop, too.

This is what was happening to Grace mid-morning. Her breakfast caused a mid-morning crash and a dip in her brain functioning. That's why it was hard for her to focus when her teacher started to go over the periodic table or explain what happens to atoms in a chemical reaction. Grace was more than smart enough to grasp the concepts in class, and she was even interested in the material, but she was working with a handicap caused by her breakfast.

Sugar, Academic Performance, and Learning Ability

Jen had $10. She spent $4.50. How much money does she have left?

This is a typical math question asked on standardized tests. It's clear and straightforward—and when kids consume too much sugar, it's less likely that they will answer it correctly.

In one of the largest and most comprehensive studies on the effects of too much sugar on academic performance, Australian researchers looked at the diets of 4,245 children ages eight to fifteen years, along with their scores on standardized, multiple-choice academic tests. The study team found that regular consumption of sugary beverages was associated with lower test scores in grammar, reading, writing, and math. As the kids consumed an increasing number of sugary beverages, their test scores got progressively worse in all four subjects. In contrast, eating vegetables at the evening meal was associated with better test scores in spelling and writing—a finding that gives parents everywhere another reason to make sure their kids eat their broccoli or green beans.

Other studies have shown that kids tend to have poorer academic performance when they have habits like eating junk food that is high in sugar, skipping breakfast, or having a sweet breakfast with processed carbohydrates and sugars, which quickly raise blood sugar. Kids with these dietary habits just don't have the steady glucose levels they need for optimum brain function. The next time your children sit down to complete a task, like coloring in a worksheet or practicing the piano, watch to see if they begin with a burst of energy that sputters out, or if they work in a steady, continuous manner. Then think back to what they ate in the hours beforehand, and you may begin to notice a pattern. Sugar changes the way children approach their tasks—and how well they finish them.

New research also shows that the effects of sugar on learning ability in children can have very early roots. A recent study followed 1,234 pregnant mothers in Boston through pregnancy and tested learning ability in their children in early childhood (around three years of age) and mid-childhood (around eight years of age). The results were striking; they showed lower test scores for standardized tests in children whose mothers consumed more sugar and sugary beverages during pregnancy. This was also the case for diet sodas; the more the expectant mothers drank during pregnancy, the poorer their children scored on tests that assessed their learning ability. In fact, this was the strongest finding from the study. This study also examined dietary patterns in the children and showed that the more sugar-sweetened beverages the children drank during early childhood, the lower they scored on verbal skills tests. While there are a number of reasons that sugar as well as alternative sweeteners could influence kids' performance on these types of tests, one important reason has to do with how sugar can impair memory.

Less Sugar, Better Memory

He studies math really hard at night, but when he takes a test the next day, it's like he's forgotten everything he learned.

I tell my sixteen-year-old that it's her responsibility to pack her own lunch in the morning, but she keeps forgetting. She does her homework, but just can't remember to take it to school, or to hand it in to the teacher. She can't even remember where she parks her car when she goes shopping! Is this normal?

Kids can be scatterbrained, and to some degree this behavior really is normal. But if your child is chronically forgetful, it's time to take a look at how much sugar they're getting. Sugar can cause amnesia-like effects, especially in the teenaged brain. In a study led by my colleague Dr. Scott Kanoski at USC, the goal was to understand whether sugar damages spatial memory, and whether the effects vary with age. In this study, rats were taught visual cues to recognize different shapes and colors. Then they were put in a maze with a harsh environment of bright lights and loud noise, which the rats did not like. In order to exit the maze, the rats had to learn and remember the visual cues that guided them to an escape hole. Imagine that you're trying to find your car in a busy and noisy mall parking lot or trying to make your way out of a chaotic high school that has many different wings and hallways, and you'll have a sense of what the rats were being asked to do.

The rats were fed their usual diet and bottle of water, but in addition, they were given either a) another bottle of water, b) a sucrose solution (table sugar), or c) a high-fructose corn syrup (HFCS) solution. The two different sugar solutions were made to mimic the concentration of a typical sugary beverage for human consumption. The rats that were given either of the sugar solutions had impaired spatial memory. They forgot their cues. They got lost more easily and couldn't escape as quickly. They finished their task more slowly than the others. Sound like any teenagers you know?

That's not all. Kanoski and his team analyzed how these sugary drinks affected the rats according to their ages, comparing adolescent rats to adult rats. It was only the adolescent rats whose memory performance was affected by consuming the sugar. Adult rats were exposed to the same sugar solutions, and they drank just as much, but there was no effect on how they performed in the tests. This damaging effect of sugar on the brain was unique to adolescent rats and not found in adults—probably because during adolescence, the brain is still developing and is more vulnerable to the damaging effects of too much sugar. When Kanoski and his team looked at the adolescent rats' brains, they found that rats drinking the sugar solutions, especially the HFCS, had inflammation in a key area of the brain called the hippocampus, which is important for memory. (People who have had damage to the hippocampus suffer from amnesia.) Giving teens too much sugar causes a hit to their brains at a critical time. What's more, this damage can be permanent. In a follow-up study, Kanoski's team went on to show that the damage to the adolescent brains lasted into adulthood, even if the rats stopped consuming sugar. Excess sugars, even if only consumed temporarily during the adolescent period, wired the brain to have permanent effects on memory.

To add insult to injury, the hippocampus also plays a role in regulating appetite. We've already talked about some of the ways sugar's effect on your blood glucose levels can make you hungry, but its effects on the hippocampus can lead to appetite problems as well. The hippocampus fields the signals that the body sends the brain to remind it of what it has eaten and tell it when it is full. When you are eating and start to feel satisfied, your gut sends messages to your brain to tell it that you have had enough. But when you eat too much sugar, those signaling pathways are obstructed, leading you to eat more. And likely to eat more sugar, given how addictive it is. It's another vicious cycle.

Sugar, memory, and appetite disruption all work together. In one large study, researchers gave students a questionnaire about their diets that asked them to recall how often, over the past year, they had consumed twenty-four common food and drink items, all of which are high in either saturated fat or refined sugar, or both (ground red meat, cooked red meat, fried chicken, salami, sausage, bacon, butter, eggs, pizza, cheese, French fries, potato chips, pancakes, pastries, cookies, cakes, ice cream, chocolate, lollipops, soft drinks, sports drinks, full-fat milk, fruit juice, white bread). In addition, two further questions assessed the frequency of added sugar usage (in cereal, tea, coffee, etc.) and frequency of eating restaurant-prepared food. The researchers then gave the students tests to assess their long-term memory. During the tests, the students listened to an audio recording of two stories and then were asked to type their recollection of the stories immediately, and then again after twenty to thirty minutes. The students who reported eating more fat and refined sugar were less likely to remember all the details that they originally recalled about the story when asked to recount it the second time. This impairment of long-term memory could help explain why some young people do poorly on tests, even when they've studied hard in the days before.

This study continued with a smaller group of students who were matched into same-gender pairs. Each pair included one student who was a high-fat and -sugar consumer and another who was a low consumer of fat and sugar, all based on their responses to the dietary questionnaire described above. None of the students was overweight. The students who had diets higher in fat and sugar fared worse on the memory tests, were less able to accurately recall what they had eaten, and also reported feeling less full than their matched pairs. This study shows that a high-sugar diet not only can affect long-term memory but also can affect eating behaviors in a way that may promote future weight gain. Considering that all of the participants in the study were of normal weight, the negative effects of having too much sugar on the brain can occur even when children are not obese, or before obesity begins to develop.

Inflammation: The Double Whammy

Now here comes a double whammy: If a person *does* become overweight, the extra body fat *itself* contributes to an inflammatory state of its own. Many people don't realize that fat is an active organ, much like your liver or your heart. It isn't just a passive blob of energy stores, but instead secretes hormones that communicate to the rest of the body, including molecules that cause inflammation. And that inflammation can *also* create memory problems.

A study conducted with overweight and obese children showed that kids with visceral adiposity, or fat around their internal organs, scored lower on tests of relational memory, or the ability to associate items. For example, the kids were asked to study pictures that showed particular animals in specific habitats. Later they were asked to recall which animals they had seen in which habitats. The researchers hypothesize that inflammation is the reason the kids with visceral fat had trouble remembering which habitat went with each animal.

When you think of inflammation, you might think of just one part of your body becoming inflamed, like the immediate area around a bite, scrape, or sprain. But inflammation can easily become systemic, or spread throughout the body, even in kids. When you have inflammation in one area, like in the case of the kids with the visceral fat, your body sends out what are called inflammatory markers to other parts of the body, including the brain. When these inflammatory factors cross the blood–brain barrier, they can cause inflammation in the brain as well. Inflammation in the brain can then cause a variety of problems, including memory impairment and loss. Although inflammation is hard to assess in human brains, new imaging techniques are beginning to make this possible. A recent study, albeit in just eleven kids, used imaging to show greater inflammation in a region of the brain called the hypothalamus that was more pronounced with increasing obesity. This is all the more relevant since the hypothalamus is the region of the brain that plays an important role in helping regulate food intake.

In summary, these impairments in memory from too much sugar can occur in normal-weight children and teens. But if a child does become overweight, the hits to his or her memory are likely to be even more pronounced because more inflammation is likely to occur in the brain.

What's the Gut Got to Do with It?

The gut (or intestines) is now actually being referred to as a "second brain." And rightly so. As a *BBC News* article explained, "There are over 100 million brain cells in your gut, as many as there are in the head of a cat." When you eat, the microorganisms that live naturally in your gut respond to what you have fed them and can produce what are called neuroactive molecules, or compounds that can send signals to your brain and regulate things like your appetite and even your mood. But sugar disrupts the balance of healthy bacteria that live in your gut by feeding the unhealthy bacteria and causing them to overpopulate. Artificial sweeteners have also been shown to disrupt gut bacteria. When your mix of gut bacteria is out of balance, the messaging between your gut and your brain is thrown off, which can lead to things like overeating and anxiety. Furthermore, we now know that eating or drinking too much sugar can weaken the lining of the gut, which can then allow toxins to pass through into the body's circulation and eventually make their way to organs like the brain, where they can affect memory, mood, and behavior.

Though we are still working to understand all of the details about the gut–brain connection, we do already know that you can promote healthy brain development in your kids and keep their memories sharp by giving them foods and drinks that foster healthy bacteria in their guts. These include high-fiber "prebiotic" foods like fruits, vegetables, legumes, and whole grains, as well as fermented "probiotic foods" like yogurt and miso.

The Crucial Skill for Success— and How Sugar Disrupts It

Does your middle schooler do her homework right after school, or does she watch YouTube for hours and then panic about her unfinished assignments?

Does your sixteen-year-old wake up late for predawn swim practice, skip the pool—and then complain that everyone else is "naturally" faster than he is?

Parents everywhere know the pain of teaching children delayed gratification, the ability to postpone a small, immediate pleasure in anticipation of a greater reward later on. It's a difficult skill but a crucial one. Young children who learn to delay gratification do better on their SATs and are described by their parents as more competent when they are teens. Studies have even shown that preschoolers who exhibit this important skill are less likely to be overweight as adults or to use drugs. They also tend to have a higher level of educational achievement, are better able to cope with stress, and have a higher sense of self-worth.

Delayed gratification is made possible through the brain's reward system, located in the prefrontal cortex. Part of the brain's reward system is the prefrontal cortex, the area of the brain that is responsible for planning and making decisions. The teenage years are especially important for the maturation of the prefrontal cortex, and adolescence is an important window for solidifying the kinds of traits that you as a parent want to encourage, such as impulse control and the ability to make smart decisions. But biology does not make this task easy. As part of normal adolescent development, teens have increased activity in the areas of the prefrontal cortex that use dopamine, a neurotransmitter that leads us to seek rewards. This is why teens are naturally more prone to thrill-seeking behaviors and acting on impulse, and are also more likely to report feeling bored. Their need for excitement is just simply higher. If you add sugar into this equation, everything intensifies. Sugar itself stimulates the release of dopamine and opioids, which can fuel these pathways and lead to an addictive cycle of more thrill seeking and sugar consumption as well to maintain high dopamine levels. In other words, sugar and the teenage brain together make a recipe for drama, and not the good kind.

While overdoing it on *any* type of sugar has harmful effects on teens, fructose has a number of its own special dangers, including its effects on the brain. A colleague at USC, Dr. Katie Page, led a study about sugar and brain activity that involved twenty-four young adults between the ages of sixteen and twenty-five. Participants were given either a glucose-based or fructose-based beverage on separate days. Each time the participants finished their drinks, the research team showed the young adults pictures of foods such as candy, cookies, pizza, and hamburgers. At the same time, they measured the participants' brain activity with an fMRI scan, which is a special magnetic resonance imaging (MRI) scan of the brain that looks at how different regions respond to certain tasks or stimulations. After drinking the fructose-based drink, the participants' brains showed greater reactivity in response to the food pictures than after they drank the glucose-based drink. When the participants drank fructose and then saw the junk foods, their brains lit up like Christmas trees. They saw those junky foods and *wanted* them, fiercely, after drinking the fructose-based beverage but not the glucose-based beverage. This study highlights what we've seen again and again: All sugar in excess is bad for kids, but fructose in particular has more damaging effects on their bodies and minds.

After the food-cue test, the researchers also gave the participants a decision-making task to complete. In this task, the participants were offered a series of choices between immediate food rewards or delayed monetary rewards based on the market value of the food items, such as cookies or pizza. The immediate food rewards included items that the participants had rated as "very attractive" on a pre-screening questionnaire. The youth were told that these foods had to be consumed right away rather than taken home. The other option was to receive a Visa gift card that would be delivered later, in an amount based on the value of the products. The results of this part of the experiment were similar to the first: After participants had the fructose drink, they were more likely to select an immediate food reward than the delayed monetary reward.

Choosing junk food now over a monetary reward later is a mild version of what poor impulse control and the inability to delay gratification look like. In real life, these traits are what lead teens to blow off studying for their finals, or skateboard down a steep hill without a helmet, or accept a dare to steal something from a convenience store, or try drugs. These studies tell us that by giving kids less sugar, and especially less fructose, we can promote the healthy development of their reward centers, and ultimately help them to make better decisions.

Longer-Term Effects: Can You Start Now to Protect Your Child from Cognitive Decline, Dementia, and Alzheimer's?

"Kids are so lucky. They can eat anything and not worry about the consequences."

Parents often use statements like the one above to justify giving their children sweet treats on a regular basis. (These parents may not realize quite how much sugar is sneaking into their kids' diets.) There's a general sense that kids get a free pass to eat whatever they want, and that only adults have to worry about the consequences of what they eat. But this "pass" doesn't exist, and it never did.

We now know that what you eat and how high your blood sugar levels are over the long term can predict your brain health during aging. A recently published study followed a group of 5,189 adults over a ten-year period and found that higher blood sugar levels were associated with cognitive decline, which refers to impairments in thinking, memory, and language. This included people who were not technically diabetic but still had elevated blood sugar levels, likely related to a diet that is high in sugar and simple carbohydrates. Research also shows that having a high-carbohydrate diet is directly linked to the development of cognitive impairment and dementia.

High blood sugar over the long term has been shown to damage an enzyme in the brain called macrophage migration inhibitory factor (MIF). This damage to MIF inhibits the ability of the brain to make glial cells. Glial cells are highly abundant in the brain. They help protect and insulate neurons and thus maintain healthy brain function. This recent discovery was made by scientists in England who analyzed the brains of people with and without Alzheimer's. They found that in the early stages of Alzheimer's, the enzyme MIF is damaged from the brain being exposed to too much sugar over time. As study author Omar Kassaar from the University of Bath in the UK explained, "Excess sugar is well known to be bad for us when it comes to diabetes and obesity, but this potential link with Alzheimer's disease is yet another reason that we should be controlling our sugar intake in our diets." That this condition develops silently over time is extremely frightening, and though we can't know exactly when the damage begins to occur, it could easily be in childhood. There's strong reason to believe that the effects of high circulating glucose in general can begin in childhood and add up over a lifetime. Alzheimer's disease is one of the most feared disorders of our time. Why not, given what we know about the harmful effects of sugar on the brain, do everything you can do protect your children now?

There is also new evidence to suggest that drinking sugar-sweetened beverages is related to signs of preclinical Alzheimer's, or the early signs that show that it is developing. The disease is characterized by plaques and tangles in the brain, nerve cell loss, tissue death, and brain shrinkage, all of which impair brain function. This analysis produced the scans that were mentioned at the beginning of this chapter, the ones showing that people who consume one to two sugary beverages a day have lower total brain volume than those who consume less than one sugary beverage a day. They also found that the higher sugar consumers scored worse on tests of episodic memory, or their unique memory of a specific event, such as what you had for dinner last night or ability to recall details of a story someone just told you twenty minutes ago. People who drank fruit juice every day experienced a similar effect, with lower total brain volume, hippocampal volume, and poorer episodic memory. This is yet another reason not to give your child sugary beverages, including juice, on a regular basis.

There are a few reasons that sugar, and especially fructose, can contribute to these serious, long-term brain issues. One has to do with brain plasticity, or the ability of the synapses (connections) in the brain to grow and change. Rats that are given a high-fructose diet for six weeks develop a variety of problems related to brain function and ability to learn. That's because fructose reduces the plasticity of their brains. When the brain loses plasticity, it ages faster and experiences declines in functioning. These changes disrupted the rats' ability to learn and also impaired their long-term memory. Other studies have shown that a high sugar diet reduces the production and functioning of brain-derived neurotrophic factor (BDNF), which is essential for long-term memory. This protein is found in several areas of the brain. It helps support the synapses and assists them in growing and changing. Reductions in BDNF have been linked to the development of dementia and Alzheimer's, as well as other conditions, including depression and schizophrenia.

At this point, you probably won't be surprised to hear us say that it's not just regular sugar that can cause long-term damage to the brain, it's low-calorie sweeteners as well. Another study showed that drinking one or more diet sodas per day is associated with a greater risk of stroke and dementia, including Alzheimer's disease. Why? Some of the most popular diet drinks, including Diet Coke, are sweetened with aspartame, which has been shown to impair memory in mice. Research has also shown that the body breaks aspartame down into various components, including phenylalanine, aspartic acid, and methanol. Phenylalanine and aspartic acid can both pass through the blood–brain barrier and are known to be toxic to the brain and contribute to memory reduction. Also, methanol can be converted by the body into formaldehyde, which can be carcinogenic and damage cellular function throughout the body. It has also been found that exposure to the sweetener AceK in mice causes abnormalities in the synapses of brain cells, resulting in impairment of memory and disruption in learning ability. A study of this sort would not be safe to conduct in humans, but these results are enough to convince us that giving AceK, or any other artificial sweeteners, to children just isn't worth the risk. Sweeteners like aspartame and AceK are found in a wide range of products such as diet beverages, baked goods, jams, yogurts, candy, and chewing gum. Also look out for them in some other healthcare products such as PediaSure nutrition drinks (marketed specifically for children and healthy growth), throat lozenges, toothpaste, vitamins, and supplements.

All this research points in one direction: If you want to help protect your children's brains from a devastating disorder later in life, begin now by reducing their sugar and sweetener intake.

> To view the scientific references cited
> in this chapter, please visit us online at
> sugarproofkids.com/bibliography.

CHAPTER FIVE

From Teeth to Toes and Everything in Between: How Sugars and Sweeteners Can Damage the Vital Parts of Growing Bodies

"She's only fourteen years old," said Arianna's mother, Laura, as she sat in our clinic's consultation room. She was quiet for a minute, trying to process the news, but then she began to sob. How could their daughter—who seemed healthy—have type 2 diabetes? Yes, Arianna had developed a little tummy since she'd stopped playing soccer the previous year. Yes, she had definitely developed a habit of drinking soda and juice every day. But Laura never suspected that her daughter was developing a chronic disease.

If your child is overweight, seems to be addicted to sweet tastes, or is suffering from fatigue, digestive problems, and other mysterious health ailments, sugar may be to blame. Sugar is reprogramming our kids' bodies, changing their metabolism and affecting the development of their internal organs. It causes disruptions that can show up in childhood or reveal themselves later in life as obesity, diabetes, heart disease, liver disease, digestive problems, asthma, and even some forms of cancer. A 2019 study that followed one hundred thousand adults in the United States over several decades found that long-term consumption of sugar is a significant factor in early mortality (death), primarily because of its links to heart disease and cancer.

When parents enroll their children in one of our clinical research studies, they are usually worried about their child's weight. But we dig deeper by taking blood samples, doing tests for diabetes, and sending kids for scans such as MRIs that can measure patterns of fat distribution around the body. Want a wake-up call for your whole family? Try hearing that your ten-year-old son has high levels of lipids (fats) in his blood showing high risk for early cardiovascular disease. Or that your twelve-year-old daughter's levels of blood glucose indicate prediabetes (one stop short of diabetes) or worse, full-blown type 2 diabetes, as was the case with Arianna. In children with sugar-related diseases, sometimes high amounts of body fat are found not only under the skin but actually surrounding the vital organs such as the heart, liver, and kidneys. Even more alarming, especially in children so young, is that it's become commonplace to see fat building up *inside* the actual organs, especially the liver. It's not just the parents of our research study participants who are scared, the kids and teens themselves are, too. An eighteen-year-old from one of our studies explained, "I am scared about the threat of diabetes. I'm scared that it runs in my family. My grandmother has it, my auntie had it, and her mother had it."

One twelve-year-old boy, William, came to us with a diagnosis of fatty liver disease. He had already had a liver biopsy, his liver enzymes were sky high, and he had been in the hospital. We examined his liver by MRI and found that his liver fat was more than three times higher than the criteria for clinical diagnosis of fatty liver disease. Almost 20 percent of his liver was composed of fat. William was at risk of decreased liver function and on track to require a new liver via a very risky liver transplant. At his first meeting with our dietician he told her he was "scared straight." He already knew that to get better he wasn't supposed to be drinking juice or soda, but in casual conversation with the dietician he let her know he was drinking lemonade with most meals—he didn't associate this in his mind as being high in sugar. He was also snacking daily on cookies.

Sugar affects a child's health, growth, and development, from head to toe, and causes a whole host of problems. Many of these problems you can't see, although there may be warning signs like weight gain. In most cases, the chronic conditions associated with high sugar develop slowly and silently and can go unnoticed. Here, you'll follow sugar molecules as they journey through the body and see how sugar affects health, growth, and development from head to toe.

Cavities and Tooth Decay: Your Dentist Was Right

A four-year-old boy named Tommy came into a pediatric dentist's clinic. His front teeth were decayed, along with his baby molars. He was sent to the hospital, where most of his teeth were extracted under general anesthesia. Tommy's parents were in the habit of giving him a bottle of flavored milk when he'd wake up too early. He'd often fall back to sleep with the bottle in his mouth, where sugar remained on his teeth. His parents had no idea that Tommy had developed what dentists call baby bottle syndrome. His teeth were completely eroded.

Parents know that sugar is the main cause of deterioration and decay of teeth, but sometimes hidden sugars can catch them by surprise. Tommy's case may sound extreme, but the number of kids experiencing severe, sugar-related dental problems is on the rise. According to the Centers for Disease Control and Prevention, tooth decay is now one of the most common chronic diseases in the United States, and by age eleven, half of all children have had a filling.

Sugar promotes the growth of certain bacteria in the mouth. These bacteria produce acid, and the acid can break down teeth, and lead to decay. Although sugar-induced tooth decay can occur at any age, infants and children are much more vulnerable for a couple of reasons.

One main reason that makes developing teeth more vulnerable to sugar is that studies have shown that the *frequency* of sugar intake can be more important to increased risk of tooth decay in developing teeth than the total amount of sugar intake. Infants and kids generally tend to eat or drink sugary foods more frequently throughout the day in between regular tooth brushing. Sippy cups encourage prolonged bouts of sucking or sipping. In addition, acidity promotes dental erosion, and popular juices and soft drinks can be very acidic. Saliva naturally protects teeth from acidic breakdown and acts as a buffer, but it can't do the job on its own. Orange juice, for example, contains citric acid or malic acid. Sodas contain either phosphoric acid or citric acid, or both. It's a perfect environment for tooth decay. Ever seen a mechanic clean the leads of a car battery with a can of Coke? Imagine that type of reaction on your toddler's new teeth.

A second reason has to do with tooth development. In adult teeth, the process of tooth decay can take an average of four years. In a child's mouth, the damage happens much faster. Fully matured teeth have a natural amount of fluoride that provides some protection, but baby teeth lack this protection. So do the newly exposed surfaces of erupting permanent teeth. This is why new teeth just coming in are much more vulnerable to the effects of extra sugars that are hanging around in your toddler's mouth.

To prevent this type of damage, avoid giving children juice or soft drinks, especially in bottles or sippy cups. Be careful with gummy candies and vitamins, which adhere to teeth. (Unfortunately, most children's vitamins contain either sugar or artificial sweeteners. To reduce damage to teeth, it is best to opt for brands that dissolve easily, rather than gummies.) Regular brushing, a lower-sugar diet, and regular dental checkups will help you keep a handle on the situation, too.

Digestion and Tummy Troubles

Growing kids can have delicate digestive systems. Upset stomachs, aching tummies, and other maladies are hallmarks of childhood. However, what you might not realize is that excessive sugar consumption may be contributing to this problem. After consumption, sugar and carbohydrates start breaking down in the mouth and are then fully broken apart into their respective components in the digestive tract. From there, those components are absorbed into the bloodstream. There are a number of ways that sugars can cause gastrointestinal problems during this digestive process:

1. The body is unable to absorb large amounts of fructose, contributing to a malabsorption problem.

2. Sugar can cause an imbalance of healthy bacteria in the gut. Over time, this imbalance can even cause a condition known as "leaky gut," which causes these bacteria to leak into the bloodstream, affecting other parts of the body.

3. Some low-calorie sweeteners (LCS) are not absorbed and affect the gut directly, causing gastrointestinal side effects like bloating, gas, and an upset tummy.

Poor Fructose Absorption

If your child is having frequent, unexplained tummy problems, one possibility is that they are reacting to excessive amounts of fructose and an inability to absorb it properly. In order to transfer glucose or fructose from the gut into the bloodstream, special transport receptors in the gut recognize these sugars and help move them into the bloodstream. Glucose is so critical to providing vital energy throughout the body that there are more than a dozen different types of transporters for glucose alone. Some are switched on with lower amounts of glucose, others with higher amounts. Either way, the body is extremely efficient at making sure glucose is absorbed from the gut so that it can be used for energy.

Fructose, on the other hand, requires another specific transporter, and there's only one type. The fructose transporter is called GLUT-5, and it isn't even present in newborns because they aren't expected to consume fructose. As children grow up and become exposed to more fructose, the gut gradually develops and turns on the body's GLUT-5 receptors. However, when the gut is bombarded by high amounts of fructose, children (and sometimes even adults) might not have enough GLUT-5 to absorb it all. If there aren't enough fructose transporters, then fructose gets stuck in the gut, where it's eaten by gut-residing bacteria. The fructose essentially ferments in the gut, and this process produces hydrogen gas or other compounds that can cause bloating and cramps. If your child suffers from chronic digestive issues, this problem, known clinically as fructose malabsorption or dietary fructose intolerance, could be a factor.

The GLUT-5 fructose transporter has a limited capacity in children by design, a sure sign that kids weren't meant to handle the amount of fructose in today's modern diet. The limit for processing a dose of fructose is typically only about 25 to 50 grams in an adult. To put that number into perspective, a single 12-ounce soda or apple juice could have around 25 grams of fructose. We don't have good data for the capacity for fructose absorption in children, but it's likely to be a much lower number, since their GLUT-5 receptors are not yet fully developed.

Scientists aren't sure why, but our ability to absorb fructose is better when there is more glucose than fructose in the sugar being absorbed. This is another reason to avoid high fructose–containing sugars like high-fructose corn syrup, agave, and fruit-based sugars. When there is more fructose than glucose, it is even harder for the fructose transporters to work well. If your child is drinking a soda made with HFCS, which could contain 65 percent fructose, you could see more tummy turmoil as a result. The same goes for apple and pear juice, which contain 70 percent fructose. Although most parents don't give their children pear juice to drink, it can be found as a sweetener in many food products—so now you have even more reason to check labels.

How to Test Your Child for Fructose Malabsorption

How can you know if your child is having trouble absorbing fructose? A pediatrician can perform a clinical test. Your child will be given a big dose of fructose, and then the doctor will collect breath samples over several hours and analyze them for hydrogen gas. If there is any malabsorption, the fructose will be fermented by the gut bacteria and produce hydrogen gas that can be measured in breath samples. However, if your child is subject to frequent bouts of gas and bloating, you can perform an easier version of this test at home. Simply try reducing sugar—especially high-fructose offenders—and see if your child feels better. In a study with 222 kids aged two to eighteen years who had unexplained abdominal issues, it turned out that more than half of the kids had fructose malabsorption after a breath test. Kids who tested positive for fructose malabsorption were advised to go on a low-fructose diet and after that, 77 percent had improvement in symptoms.

Your Child's Gut Microbiome: A Key to Digestion, Mood, and Memory

Inside your digestive system, trillions of microorganisms live and thrive The exact composition of this world-within-world, known as your microbiome, is unique to you. It's made up mostly of bacteria, though viruses and yeasts can also be found. Some of these bacteria are helpful and play an important role in keeping you healthy, while others might produce harmful compounds. We aren't born with our microbiome. Instead, it's established in the first few years of life, which means that a child's early life exposures can shape the eventual profile of the microbiome. How a child is born (vaginal birth versus C-section) and fed (breastfeeding versus formula) can have major effects.

The microbiome is a relatively new field of study. But there are studies under way, including in my lab, to advance our understanding of how early nutrition affects microbiome development. We want to know more about how exposure to sugar during early microbiome development in infancy could play a role and shape later health, from a child's predisposition to diabetes and obesity to brain health. It's a new field of research, and studies take time. We have to take frequent measures of diet in childhood (including analysis of breast milk so we know its exact composition), collect frequent samples of stool from the infants to determine how the gut microbiome is evolving, and follow the kids for long enough into early childhood to be able to determine outcomes like cognitive ability.

While we wait for these human studies to complete, we're gathering some initial clues from studies in lab rats. These studies can be performed faster than studies of humans, and it's easier to tightly control the conditions. Dr. Scott Kanoski, who has been conducting the studies of sugar and memory that we've described earlier, also studies the effects of sugar on the gut. In one of his studies, Scott gave rats access to their normal food, along with a choice of beverages: plain drinking water or an 11 percent solution of sugar, which mimics sugary beverages. A control group received just their normal food and water. Naturally, the rats with access to the sugar water chose to drink it—and Scott found that this group had major disruptions to their microbiome, with more harmful bacteria present. This imbalance may have effects beyond the digestive system because gut bacteria can produce neuroactive molecules. These molecules can send signals to the brain along a line of communication known as the gut–brain axis. When the gut–bacteria balance isn't properly calibrated, it can short-circuit this communication, altering your appetite, mood, and brain function, as we talked about in the last chapter. In follow-up studies, Scott is now examining whether the sugar-induced disruption in the gut microbiome contributes to the brain- and memory-related impairments.

Too much sugar can lead to other problems with gut bacteria. When these bacteria leak into the circulatory system, the result is a disorder called intestinal permeability, also known as leaky gut. Leaky gut causes everything from diarrhea and constipation to headache and fatigue and liver problems. Fructose in particular has been linked to leaky gut, and leaky gut has been shown to be a factor contributing to diseases like type 2 diabetes and cardiovascular disease. If you want to protect your child's digestive system, make it a priority to avoid fruit juice and products sweetened with juice, high-fructose corn syrup, agave, fruit sugar, and fruit juice concentrates, all of which are high in fructose.

Low-Calorie Sweeteners (LCS) and GI Problems

It's not just regular sugars that can cause gastrointestinal distress. Low-calorie sweeteners (LCS) can also cause intestinal problems. Remember Melissa, the soccer-playing girl from the beginning of this book who suffered from fatigue and stomach cramps? Melissa had been chewing several sticks of sugar-free gum each day. When she gave up her gum habit, her stomach cramps improved.

Kids and adults alike chew sugar-free gum in the hopes of avoiding cavities, but take a close look at the labels. You might see warnings about potential digestive side effects, especially when products contain sugar alcohols like sorbitol or xylitol. Some of them even have effects similar to laxatives. Sugar alcohols aren't broken down in the small intestine and can cause water retention, stomach cramps, and discomfort—and in the worst cases, even dehydration and diarrhea. Other LCS, including stevia, sucralose, and saccharin, are not absorbed into the bloodstream. These LCS that aren't absorbed or broken down can build up in the gut where they can affect the normal composition of the gut microbiome.

Fatty Liver Disease: The New Kid in Town

The liver is a workhorse organ. You might take it for granted, but you shouldn't. Everything that is absorbed into the bloodstream from the food and drinks that we consume, immediately passes through the liver, which acts like a giant filter. It recognizes toxins and clears them from the blood. You really don't want anything to interfere with this critically important filtering system. But that's exactly what happens in nonalcoholic fatty liver disease (NAFLD), which is another term for buildup of fat in the liver. Over time, NAFLD can result in major health problems and even require a liver transplant.

Thirty years ago, no one had even heard of NAFLD. It wasn't even a diagnostic condition. Most people think of fatty liver disease as something alcoholics suffer from—not children. Alcohol is also processed by the liver, where it is converted to fat through a very similar process as fructose, which is why fructose has been referred to as "alcohol without the buzz." However, in today's new food environment, the nonalcoholic form of fatty liver disease is now the most common type and is becoming an epidemic, even in children, and a common reason for liver transplants. On very few doctors' radars until recently, it can be hard to diagnose. NAFLD is a silent disease, meaning that even if your child has it, you wouldn't know it until your child experiences moderate to severe abdominal pain and a yellowing coloring of the eyes and skin—and at that point, the disease would be advanced. It may only be diagnosed in passing when a child is examined for other health problems. If routine blood tests reveal elevated liver enzymes, the doctor may go on to confirm the diagnosis with an ultrasound and eventually a liver biopsy.

A biopsy can be risky, and without their child showing symptoms, many parents understandably don't want to take that risk. Because of this it is difficult to know the true extent of this problem. However, a study in 2006 got around this problem by examining the livers from hundreds of children who had died of various accidental causes and found that 13 *percent* of all children met the clinical criteria for fatty liver. Among children who were obese, 38 percent had a fatty liver. This finding launched major new clinical and research initiatives to help understand the reasons for its early onset in childhood, how better to diagnose it, and how to treat and prevent it.

In 2007, one of my colleagues at Children's Hospital Los Angeles, Dr. Rohit Kohli, started one of the first specialty clinics to treat kids with fatty liver disease. He has treated patients as young as five years old, although the typical age of his patients is nine or older. When he first opened his clinic in Cincinnati before coming to Los Angeles, none of the parents of these children had even heard of the disease. Within a few years, families had heard a bit more about it, or maybe they had a spouse or sibling who had it, but they didn't know it existed in children. Now he finds parents are beginning to understand that NAFLD is a real problem for some children today, and he refers to fatty liver disease as the "silent tsunami."

In 2013, Jean Welsh, an epidemiologist at the Centers for Disease Control and Prevention, came up with a simple assessment for what she calls "suspected fatty liver disease" based on measures of liver enzymes in blood and weight status. Jean used data from large national surveys that were completed during different time periods, allowing her to examine trends over time. Between the early 1990s to 2010, a period of less than twenty years, cases of suspected fatty liver disease in children more than doubled, from 4 percent to 11 percent. What's more, about half of all kids who were overweight had suspected NAFLD and didn't even know it.

Sugar, especially the rise in fructose consumption, is behind this dramatic new reality. The liver converts fructose into fat in a process called *de novo lipogenesis*, which means "new fat synthesis." This new fat can either become trapped in the liver or released into the blood for transport around the body. Both of these outcomes cause problems. If these newly synthesized fats find their way into the bloodstream, the long-term risk of heart disease increases—more on that later. And if the fat ends up in the liver, and if enough fat is trapped there over time, the liver will no longer be able to do its job of clearing toxins from the blood. Those toxins will do damage to the body. Damage to the liver is progressive, resulting eventually in liver cancer. Moreover, liver fat is probably the worst kind of fat you can have in terms of increasing the risk for type 2 diabetes. As pediatric endocrinologist Robert Lustig at the University of California, San Francisco, has said, "We are turning our children's livers into foie gras."

The good news is that we can reverse NAFLD in kids simply by changing their diets. Stripping added sugars out of the diet can have fairly rapid effects on reducing fat buildup in the liver. In a randomized trial, forty boys with NAFLD were given a diet that was very low in added sugars. When we say "very low," we mean it: The goal was to get sugar down to only 3 percent of total daily calories. A control group of boys continued their high-sugar diets. After eight weeks, the low-sugar group saw success, with their liver fat reduced from an average of 25 percent of liver mass to 17 percent. The control group showed no change. How reproducible are these findings in real life? Well, the diet was fairly extreme for these kids to follow, and they were given lots of help by the research team, which prepared foods for them.

We have an ongoing study that also has a focus on reducing sugar out of the diet to treat children with fatty liver disease and shows that this approach can work in real life situations. Rosa, a seventeen-year-old girl, was referred to our study after she received a diagnosis of NAFLD and, like William, was, as she put it, "scared straight." After meeting with our dietician several times over the course of twelve weeks, both of these kids were able to make subtle but effective changes in their diets. For example, William readily gave up his lemonade drinks for regular or unsweetened, flavored water once he realized they were so high in sugar. A typical breakfast for Rosa before the intervention was white bread with jam or sweetened breakfast cereal with milk and a banana. By the end of the study, her typical breakfast was egg whites on whole-wheat toast. These dietary changes weren't nearly as drastic as the ones in the study of forty boys, but they still had positive effects. Even though she gained a little bit of weight during her time in our program (probably because she was still growing), Rosa felt like she was losing weight because her clothes were fitting her better. Rosa's blood cholesterol improved, and, more remarkable, her liver fat fell from 13.3 percent to 5.9 percent, leaving her only slightly above the clinical criteria for NAFLD. As for William, he also made a dramatic improvement with significant reductions in his liver enzymes, a drop in his liver fat to below the clinical threshold, and improvements in his cholesterol and blood pressure. Our hope is that kids like Rosa and William can continue to make and sustain small changes—and continue to improve their liver health.

Other Risk Factors for Fatty Liver

You may be wondering if your own child is at risk for liver disease. In general, boys and men are more prone to the disease, as are people who are overweight. Another risk factor is poor early nutrition, including in utero. In a study performed on primates, liver fat was almost five times higher in offspring born to mothers who were fed a high-fat/high-sugar diet during pregnancy. Remarkably, this higher liver fat was present even before birth in the developing fetus. We can't measure fetal liver fat in humans; however, we can check it immediately after birth with an MRI scan. In one study, babies born to mothers who were overweight had liver fat that was 68 percent higher than babies born to mothers who were normal weight. How could this happen? While a baby is still developing in the womb, fat cells are not yet fully developed. And in infancy, those same fat cells are undergoing very rapid growth. When fat cells are either not developed or aren't available to store excess calories, fat is stored in other places in the body, such as the liver.

Some ethnic groups are particularly prone to accumulating large amounts of fat in the liver. Compared to Caucasians, for example, Hispanics are more likely to have higher buildups of fat, and African Americans are much less likely to have high liver fat accumulation. A particular gene that interferes with the breakdown and release of fat from the liver—called PNPLA3—is found in half of all Hispanics, compared to only about 10 percent of African Americans and Caucasians. A large study in 2008 found that the gene is associated with having twice as much fat in the liver. In our studies in Hispanic children, we have found that the effect of this gene on liver fat was manifested as young as eight years of age. (We think that this could be evident even earlier in life, but liver fat is measured via an MRI, a procedure that is challenging for young children to complete as they have to lie still for about half an hour, so we haven't done studies in younger children.) Also, we found that consuming high amounts of sugar exacerbated the effect of the PNPLA3 gene on liver fat. In other words, the effect of this gene is turned on by a high-sugar diet. If your family is Hispanic, you may want to pay extra attention to your children's risk for liver disease.

Diabetes: Sugar and the Pancreas

If you want to understand diabetes, begin with insulin. Insulin is produced by the pancreas, within specialized cells called beta cells. The production and release of insulin is critical to getting glucose from your blood into the parts of the body that need it for energy like your muscles or your brain. In most people this is a very tightly controlled process, what we call homeostatic regulation. Think of the thermostat that controls the temperature where you live. When the temperature (blood glucose) falls, the furnace (beta cells in the pancreas) turns on and pumps out more heat (insulin). When the specified temperature is reached, the furnace turns off. If the pancreas can't produce insulin, or can't product enough of it, then too much glucose builds up in the blood, eventually resulting in the symptoms of diabetes. We don't want to scare you, but there is a reasonable chance your child will experience these symptoms: One out of every three kids growing up today will develop diabetes at some point in their lives. For Hispanics, the outlook is even worse, with one in two predicted to get the disease.

When we talk about diabetes in this book, we're talking about type 2 diabetes. This form of diabetes was unheard of in children until about twenty years ago. We first saw reports of it in children in the year 2000. Now, five thousand new cases are diagnosed in children each year. Type 2 diabetes begins as a condition known as insulin resistance. In its initial stages, the pancreas is still able to make insulin—but either the body can't make enough of it, or the body doesn't respond properly to the insulin it does produce. Eating too much sugar can contribute to this problem, because the pancreas has to release extra insulin every time sugar comes into the body. This continuously high level of insulin causes the body's cells to become resistant to insulin. They are hesitant to open the gates when insulin tries to unlock them so that glucose can enter. The pancreas has to pump out more insulin in order to clear glucose from the bloodstream.

If the body keeps receiving high doses of sugar and carbohydrates, the situation will worsen. The pancreas has to work harder and harder, and as it becomes more difficult for your body to clear glucose from your blood, your levels of blood glucose can rise to a point known as prediabetes. Estimates suggest that one in three adults in the United States have prediabetes and that 90 percent of those adults don't even know they have it. Estimates of prediabetes in US children are not well established, although some of our studies indicate that about 40 percent of overweight or obese children already have prediabetes.

Over time, the constant and continual demand for more and more insulin eventually wears down the ability of the pancreas to produce enough insulin to cope with the glucose onslaught. That's when type 2 diabetes occurs. To come back to the central heating analogy: Imagine that your temperature sensors aren't working or that you left the back door open, so your furnace just keeps pumping out more and more heat. Eventually your furnace wears down and grinds to a halt. But in your body, this system failure doesn't happen overnight. Type 2 diabetes is a silent and slowly progressing disease that might go undiagnosed for some time. All the while, the high levels of blood glucose contribute to disorders like kidney disease, heart disease, and nerve damage. Because of these complications, diabetes is the seventh leading cause of death in the United States.

The Goran lab has been researching factors that affect diabetes risk in children and teens for more than twenty-five years. In 2002, I received a major grant from the National Institutes of Health that made it possible to start a long-term study—one that ran for the next fifteen years. We recruited a group of 250 children who were at a high risk for developing type 2 diabetes. Each year, we took measurements of diet and body fat; we performed blood tests and scans to measure diabetes risk. When I started the study, I wasn't totally focused on diet because I wasn't convinced it could be measured accurately enough in children. It is hard for kids to remember what they eat. You have to rely on parents to help them recall, but that itself is difficult, as kids are at school and away from their parents for part of the day.

Then, in 2005, Jaimie Davis, a newly graduated PhD who is also a registered dietician, came to work in my lab. Jaimie is so energetic that she would literally do back flips at lab meetings when good news was announced. Always chirpy and upbeat, Jaimie convinced the lab to place more focus on carefully assessing diet as best we could, and to relate these assessments to children's risk for diabetes. During this time, Emily was also working in the lab as a study coordinator and nutrition educator, and later as a graduate student. Together, over the next ten years, we produced more than a dozen scientific papers looking at how dietary factors affected development of diabetes and metabolic risk in these children. We were looking at dietary factors in general, not just sugar, but a clear pattern emerged that implicated dietary sugar in kids' risk for diabetes. Our first major paper showed a relationship between sugary beverage intake in Hispanic kids and the ability of their beta cells in the pancreas to produce enough insulin to keep their blood glucose in check. Since then, a consistent pattern has emerged. Almost all studies, not just the ones from our lab, show that higher consumption of sugar, especially in the form of sugary beverages, increases the risk of developing type 2 diabetes. Depending on how much sugar children are consuming, their diabetes risk can jump up by 18 to 26 percent.

What about the sugar in juice and fruit? In a very large study that followed almost two hundred thousand adults over time, epidemiologists found that drinking fruit juice increases the risk of diabetes by about 10 percent. The same scientists looked at whole fruit and found that some fruits lowered risk, while others increased it. Blueberries in particular were the most protective, with three servings per week reducing risk for diabetes by 25 percent. Other fruits were also found to be protective—for example, three servings per week of grapes, apples, or pears reduced risk by 12 percent and 7 percent, a fact that might be surprising, given that these fruits are higher in fructose. It's possible that their fructose content might be offset by the fiber and other protective phytochemicals in these fruits, which is another reason to eat fruit rather than drink it. In contrast, cantaloupe increased risk by about 10 percent, perhaps because its sugar is quickly absorbed into the bloodstream. Also interesting is that some health professionals have recommended fructose as a sugar of choice for diabetics, because the body does not use insulin to process it. Using fructose alone will avoid the need for insulin and lead to better control of blood glucose. But it may then cause its own set of serious problems, including liver disease.

Alternative sugars and LCS don't always offer diabetics better options, either. Physicians and dietitians often recommend LCS products to diabetics as sugar substitutes, but a study conducted in youth with type 1 diabetes found that diabetic kids who consumed higher levels of LCS beverages actually had higher blood glucose levels as well as increased levels of cholesterol. Some of the kids who used LCS in this study had an overall lower-quality diet, which could have contributed to high blood glucose from simple carbohydrates or other processed foods. However, other research in nondiabetic kids and adults confirms that using LCS actually leads to worse control of blood sugar. Other studies in adults support the idea that LCS and sucralose in particular may promote higher blood glucose levels and overproduction of insulin. It may be that sucralose can trick the body into thinking it's consumed actual sugar.

Insulin Resistance in Adolescence: Why Teenagers Are Especially at Risk

One important factor contributes to insulin resistance and risk for type 2 diabetes that's relevant to *all* children: adolescence. In 2001, we reported results from one of our studies that followed a group of kids for up to twelve years and brought them to the lab for testing at different stages of puberty. All kids, regardless of gender, ethnicity, or weight status, became about 30 percent more insulin resistant in the middle of puberty. We're still not sure why this occurs, but it means that the beta cells in the pancreas have to work extra hard during puberty to produce enough insulin to clear glucose from the circulation, regardless of diet or body weight status. Therefore, teens should be especially careful to consume a healthy, low-sugar diet so that their beta cells don't get overworked. This helps lower their risk for insulin resistance, prediabetes, and type 2 diabetes.

Heart Disease

We've been led to believe that fat in the diet is the main dietary cause of heart disease, a belief that's still taught in some nutrition classes. So you might not think of sugar as an obvious cause. In the 1960s and '70s, the food industry wanted to dispel the belief that sugar contributed to heart disease. Low-fat diets were becoming more popular, and the food industry started producing more processed low-fat food options. What made them taste good? Sugar. And of course, the sugar industry was eager to influence public opinion away from sugar's possible harmful effects. Cristin Kearns, a professor at the University of California, San Francisco School of Dentistry, discovered troves of historical documents on sugar-related research and found that trade groups paid top scientists at places like Harvard to publish influential papers and commentaries to downplay sugar's hazardous effects. They wanted to point the blame at fat and shelve studies that found damaging effects of sugars.

Now that unbiased scientists have conducted new studies, we understand more about how various sugars are processed by the body and contribute to the risk of heart disease. An overdose of sugar won't cause your child to collapse from a heart attack, but just like fatty liver disease and diabetes, heart disease develops slowly and silently, often with no outward signs.

A classic study in 1992 examined 150 kids who had died accidentally. The study found that even in children without any clinical signs of heart disease before death, fatty streaks were already building up in their aortas. Some of these children had undergone blood testing prior to their deaths; the higher their blood cholesterol, the more likely they were to have fatty streaks. Collectively, these findings show that cardiovascular disease development can begin in childhood and that the early measurement of blood cholesterol could be a useful prognostic indicator.

One of the largest and clearest studies linking sugar to heart disease was published by researchers at Harvard in 2014. They followed more than ten thousand men and women in the United States between

1988 and 2006, and they discovered that people who had consumed more sugar had a higher risk of death from heart disease. Compared to a reference group that consumed less than 10 percent of calories from added sugars, those consuming 10 to 25 percent of daily calories from added sugars had a 30 percent increase in death. In people who consumed more than 25 percent of their daily calories from added sugar, the risk of death from heart disease was almost three times higher.

Getting 25 percent of your daily calories from added sugar might sound like a lot to you, and it is. For adults, it's the equivalent of drinking three cans of full-sugar soda each day (assuming that was the only source of added sugar). But this level of sugar consumption is actually pretty common among kids. According to a study that tracked eight thousand kids between the ages of two and eighteen, the average sugar intake is 118 grams per day—or 25 percent of all calories. Sugar consumption was highest in kids ages two to five (28 percent of calories from sugar) compared to teens (24 percent of calories). What does this mean? Put simply, the average child is consuming the same percentage of sugar per day as adults who are three times more likely to die from heart disease.

How does increased sugar cause heart disease? We know that increased sugar intake contributes to obesity, which by itself is known to increase the risk of heart disease. However, studies also show that increased sugar intake can cause additional effects on heart disease, beyond the effects of the calories. This is because of the way sugar is metabolized, or broken down, by the body. This is especially true for fructose. Remember how fructose is processed in the liver and converted to fat? This newly synthesized fat can be stored in the liver, but most of it gets repackaged into other types of fat-containing molecules suitable for transportation in blood. This transportable fat increases blood cholesterol levels and likes to adhere in all sorts of places in the body—including the blood vessels around the heart. It is the buildup of these molecules in blood that contributes to long-term heart disease.

Dr. Kimber Stanhope, a sugar researcher at the University of California, Davis, has dedicated the last few decades of her career to demonstrating the link between sugar and heart disease. Kimber and her team have conducted a series of meticulous studies in which diets of varying sugar content were prepared and given to healthy adult volunteers living under carefully controlled conditions. These studies clearly showed that it was excess fructose in the diet, but not excess glucose, that caused significant worsening of risk factors for cardiovascular disease, and that the more fructose that was given to the test subjects, the worse the effects on cardiovascular risk. In fact, participants showed noticeable cardiovascular deterioration after just two weeks on the high-fructose test diets. But glucose did not lead to an increase in risk.

Fructose can also contribute to heart disease by raising blood pressure. Your blood vessels need nitric oxide; it helps them relax with the ebb and flow of circulation. But fructose lowers nitric oxide production in blood vessels. Because blood vessels become more rigid as fatty plaques are deposited, blood pressure rises as a demand for more circulation occurs. Uric acid can also raise blood pressure—and guess what produces uric acid when it's processed by the body? Fructose. Finally, excess fructose can cause the kidneys to retain salt in the body rather than excrete it. The combined impact of these factors on blood pressure can in turn cause hypertension and stress on the heart muscle.

The good news? You can dramatically reduce your child's risk of developing heart disease by rightsizing their sugar intake now.

Obesity

Obesity in kids is a difficult issue to tackle. Some parents work hard to preserve their children's self-esteem, telling them there's nothing wrong with being overweight. Others know that obesity is a health danger but find putting their kids on a "diet" to be heartbreaking. Worse, some are in complete denial, adamant that their kids will grow out of it. In the realm of children's health issues, obesity is probably the most challenging to fix. Nothing seems to work very well, and it is affecting younger and younger patients all the time.

Dr. Alaina Vidmar, one of my colleagues at Children's Hospital Los Angeles, receives all the obesity referrals. Her patients range from six months to eighteen years old, with plenty of children in the astonishingly young age range of twelve to twenty-four months. Typically, the first thing she hears from parents is that they "have no idea" why they have been referred to an expert in obesity. They've usually received a referral from a concerned pediatrician, but the parents are usually convinced that their child will "grow into their weight." It can be hard to get children and families to take the situation seriously. Dr. Rohit Kohli, the fatty liver specialist at Children's Hospital who was introduced earlier, recalls seeing a nine-year-old boy who weighed 210 pounds. The boy asked, "Can you just give me a pill to fix this?"

Although obesity is now considered a disease in its own right, it remains a difficult topic to talk to families about. Dr. Kohli has learned what *not* to say to families. One of his patients was an obese seven-year-old boy who also had fatty liver disease, so he decided it was time to talk to the parents about the underlying issue: their child's weight. The mom and dad, who were both obese, blew up and stormed out of the consulting room, denying that their kid had a weight problem. It's a delicate issue, but this denial puts kids at increased risk for a whole host of health issues including diabetes, fatty liver disease, cardiovascular disease, cancer, and more. Because of the severity of the situation, physicians like Dr. Kohli feel compelled to be straightforward with patients and their families even though they try to be as tactful as possible. Research shows that the earlier a child has a high-sugar diet, the more likely the child is to become obese. Sugar is what we call a modifiable risk, which means it can be controlled, so having these early conversations is critical to a child's health.

My research team conducted a study in schoolkids from economically deprived parts of Los Angeles and found that they were up to seven times more likely to be obese than kids from more affluent neighborhoods. These study results provided one of the first and clearest examples of such a striking economic difference in children. To continue this line of investigation, we next looked into what types of modifiable factors might explain this big difference. We found that among kids from lower-income families, a major factor explaining differences in obesity prevalence by two to four years of age is the number of sugary beverages they drink. Even at this young age there was a clear difference in obesity that lined up with beverage habits. Children who were not yet drinking any sugary beverages had an obesity rate of 14 percent. Kids who drank one sugary beverage per day had a rate of 18 percent. Those who had two or more sugary beverages per day had the highest rate of obesity, at 24 percent.

No matter what your family's income level or ethnic background, sugary beverages are dangerous for your kids. A year after our research was published, a study of ten thousand children from across the United States showed a clear relationship between sugary beverages and early onset of obesity. They found that children who were regular consumers of sugary beverages at two years of age had a much bigger increase in body weight over the following two years. This study also showed that toddlers who regularly drank 100 percent juice had a 30 percent higher risk of becoming overweight over the following two years. In 2014, a study by the CDC that tracked infants and children from across the United States over a long period of time showed that the earlier sugar is introduced to children in the first year of life, the greater the risk of obesity by age six.

The collective findings from these studies is clear: the earlier you introduce sugar into your child's diet, the greater the risk to your child's current and future health. We think this effect is related to the way young children's bodies undergo development. Their little bodies are rapidly building all types of cells, including fat cells. Premature fat cells, known as preadipocytes, are abundant in both infants and toddlers. Even very low amounts of sugar, especially fructose, can dramatically alter the fate of these cells. Even a very low amount of fructose can turn on a gene responsible for increased growth of fat cells, which creates a bigger fat mass.

The risk of weight gain and obesity in children can begin even earlier, during pregnancy—if a mother consumes a lot of sugar. Regardless of how the sugar is delivered—via regular sugar or sugar-sweetened beverages or food that breaks down into sugar—it affects developing cells. Both glucose and fructose can cross the placenta to reach the baby in the womb. Babies' premature fat cells are probably growing more rapidly than they will after birth, which means they can be even more susceptible to the reprogramming effects of sugar. And glucose that makes its way to the fetus can cause production of extra insulin, which can lead to extra fat storage.

Low-calorie sweeteners used during pregnancy may have the same effect. Consuming LCS during pregnancy can double an unborn child's risk of becoming overweight or obese later in life. We don't understand all the reasons for this effect, but one reason is clear. Just like fructose, LCS (saccharin and AceK, for example) can trigger the development of more and bigger fat cells. Also, new animal studies show that maternal consumption of LCS during pregnancy and lactation can have major effects on disrupting offspring gut microbiome and metabolism in ways that can contribute to metabolic diseases—even when the actual exposure in the offspring is very small. We believe this is a reason for serious concern, given that LCS consumption in pregnant women in the United States has increased from 16 percent (in 1999–2004) to 24 percent of women in 2007–2014. The biggest consumers are non-Hispanic white and educated women.

From Aches to Asthma: Mystery Illnesses

"My ankles hurt."

"It's hard to breathe when I run."

Parents who are looking for the causes of mystery ailments should consider whether inflammation plays a role. Inflammation, which is what happens when your body triggers an immune response, can become chronic and spread throughout the body. We've already talked about the way sugar leads to systemic inflammation, which in turn can affect the brain and memory. Systemic inflammation can also play a role in a host of other disorders, including asthma, joint pain, and even heart disease, stroke, and cancer.

If your child suffers from asthma, take a look at their diet. A large study of almost two thousand children found that kids who drink more than five sugary beverages a week are five times more likely to develop asthma than kids who drink less than one per month. There is also evidence to suggest that a higher intake of sugar during pregnancy is related to an increased risk of asthma for the child. Why would sugar intake lead to asthma? Because sugar increases inflammation, and asthma is an inflammatory condition. Dietary sugar, especially from beverages, is associated with a generalized inflammatory state. This type of inflammation can be measured by testing circulating levels of C-reactive protein, or CRP. If you drink sugary beverages on a daily basis, your CRP can shoot up between 60 and 100 percent.

Another ailment that is connected to inflammation is gout. You might think of gout as a disease caused by eating too much meat or drinking too much alcohol. But sugar, and specifically fructose, can also trigger this inflammatory condition. The pain and inflammation of gout is caused by deposits of uric acid crystals in the joints. And, recall from the section on blood pressure, that this uric acid is produced as a by-product from the way fructose is broken down in the liver. One of the most consistent findings associated with increased consumption of sugars, and especially sugary beverages, is an increase in circulating levels of uric acid. This is so consistent that some researchers consider using uric acid levels in blood as an independent marker of sugary beverage consumption. An analysis of ten different studies concluded that sugary beverage consumption was associated with a 35 percent increase in risk for increased uric acid and gout. And in detailed feeding studies, an increase in uric acid was due to increased fructose in particular. Usually, uric acid is filtered out by the kidneys, but when levels become too high, the uric acid can crystallize and be deposited in the joints of the extremities of the body such as fingers, toes, and ankles. The result is a sharply painful sensation.

Not long after I moved to Los Angeles in 1999, I (Michael) started to experience sudden flare-ups of red, painful inflammation in my toes and ankles. After several trips to the doctor, I was diagnosed with gout. I wanted to find the source, and tracing it took a while. I eventually figured it out one day after stopping at one of the fruit vendors on the Health Science Campus at USC. The vendors there sell big, beautiful bags of fresh, chopped fruits, like mango, watermelon, cantaloupe, and pineapple, with the optional addition of fresh lime and chili powder. On occasion I'd buy a bag for lunch. On this particular day I noticed that within hours of eating it, I had a flare-up in my ankles. That's when the light bulb went on and I made the connection between fructose and gout. This story is in no way intended to put you off fruit. I still enjoy two to three servings of fruit spread out over the day without any problems. We wholeheartedly encourage you to do the same. Just watch out for eating too much fruit all at once.

If your kids have asthma, or if they complain of achy joints in the hands, feet, or ankles, or if they simply suffer from mysterious symptoms, try skipping soda and juice for a few days, or back off of very large servings of fruit. It's still important to follow the doctor's prescription for any medication or other treatments. But if eliminating soda and juice helps your kids feel better, you've got a powerful clue as to a possible contributing factor: inflammation.

The Sugar Roller Coaster, Menstruation, and Fertility

Sugar can contribute to menstrual irregularities. Polycystic ovarian syndrome (PCOS) affects an estimated one in ten women and causes hormonal imbalances, including elevated insulin. It can cause insulin resistance and irregular periods, both of which can be tough for a teenage girl. Later in life, it can cause difficulty conceiving. I (Emily) know about PCOS firsthand, as I was diagnosed with it as a teen. In my teens and early twenties, I spent a lot of time on the sugar roller coaster. I suffered from frequent episodes of low blood sugar, which I later learned were connected to elevated insulin levels caused by PCOS. While working toward my master's degree in public health nutrition in my late twenties, I learned how to maintain a diet that is low on the glycemic index. For example, I used to eat a high-carbohydrate breakfast, such as oatmeal with fruit or whole-grain cereal with a plant-based milk. Now I know that I can't tolerate that type of carbohydrate load, especially in the morning. Within an hour of eating that way, I am irritable, hungry again, and sometimes even shaky. Now I usually have eggs with avocado and vegetables, sometimes with a small piece of toast, but often with salad greens instead. Since I have changed my breakfast and am careful to pair carbohydrates with protein and healthy fat at other times in the day as well, I only rarely have a blood sugar emergency. Despite being told by multiple specialists that I would have a hard time getting pregnant, I was able to regulate my periods through diet and exercise alone, and had both of my boys without needing fertility treatments. Research validates my experience that carefully managing carbohydrate intake can reduce PCOS symptoms.

For a Clearer Complexion, Nix the Sodas

There is a lot of speculation about the possible links between diet and acne. Some say chocolate is a trigger; others blame the oil from fried foods. We know that acne is related to hormones, which is why it flares up in the teenage years. The reality is that there hasn't been a whole lot of research on diet and acne, but studies show that sugar can be a contributor. For example, a large study of Chinese teenagers found that daily soft drink consumption significantly increases the risk of moderate to severe acne. In a study of 139 sets of twins, the twin with higher sugar intake had more acne. The twin study is especially interesting because it controls for the influence of genetics, which may also influence one's skin. Other research suggests that a number of dietary factors are related to acne, including added sugar, total sugar, foods that are high on the glycemic index, number of milk servings per day, saturated fat and trans-fatty acids, and fewer servings of fish per day. The message is clear: Your child's overall diet quality can make a difference for their skin health, and sugar plays a role. (Rosa, the teen who cut back on sugar and reduced the fat in her liver, reported that her acne cleared up, too.) In fact, a low-glycemic diet appears to reduce acne, with a significant improvement in skin lesions. A low-glycemic diet reduces insulin demand, which reduces levels of androgens and sebum production, which are the main culprits behind acne.

Can Sugar Accelerate Cellular Aging?

Telomeres, the part of the chromosomes that protect the structure of our DNA, are markers for cellular aging. They gradually deteriorate with age—and now we know that lifestyle factors such as stress and diet can accelerate this deterioration, leading to general aging and cancer risk. Some preliminary studies have shown a link between high sugary beverage consumption and shrinkage of telomere length, and one provocative study in a small sample of children showed that this shrinkage can already start to happen in the first few years of life.

Cancer

Of all diseases, cancer probably strikes the most fear into a parent's heart. And while we aren't trying to say that if your kids eat too much sugar they're going to get cancer, we do think it's fair to let you know there is an accumulating body of evidence that suggests that too much sugar can contribute to increased lifelong risk of cancer. It's hard to develop high-quality research that can carefully investigate this suggestion. We are not aware of any studies that have examined links between sugars in childhood and cancer in adulthood. But many studies have looked at a connection between sugar and cancer in adults.

One large analysis found that fructose in particular was significantly associated with increased lifelong risk of pancreatic cancer. For each 25 grams (6¼ teaspoons) of fructose per day, the risk of pancreatic cancer increased by 22 percent. This effect was fairly consistent across five out of the six studies analyzed. Another report pooled results across fourteen different studies and showed a 20 percent risk of pancreatic cancer due to carbonated sugary beverage intake. In another very large study in Australia in just over thirty-five thousand adults, increased intake of sugary beverages (more than one per day) increased risk of all obesity-related cancers (for example, colon cancer, postmenopausal breast cancer, and prostate cancer) by 18 percent. While there is currently no evidence to suggest that sugars are a cause for childhood cancer specifically, ongoing studies in both children and adults are examining whether reducing sugars and calories in general might help make chemotherapy more successful.

The reasons that too much sugar may put anyone at risk for cancer are not clear. The old way of thinking is that too much sugar directly fuels cancer cells to grow. This idea is too simplistic and probably not true. Another possibility is related to insulin. As extra glucose is consumed, more insulin is produced. And higher levels of insulin are related to a number of other similar hormones, including insulin-like growth factors (IGFs). It's possible that this environment of higher insulin and IGF promotes both cell growth and cancer. And new research is showing that cancer cells process glucose for energy in a way that's different from regular cells, and this process can activate certain proteins that interfere with regular cellular growth.

No matter *how* sugar might cause cancer, it's wise to keep kids from indulging in too much. And in general, if you Sugarproof your kids you can help them reverse or avoid a series of disorders, from diabetes to obesity to heart disease. In the next part of this book, we'll show you how.

To view the scientific references cited in this chapter, please visit us online at sugarproofkids.com/bibliography.

Part Two

Sugarproof Your Child...and Your Family

CHAPTER SIX

Sweet Talk: Motivate Your Family for Success

Now that you have a sense of sugar's very real and often hidden dangers, you can tackle the job to Sugarproof your kids. Being Sugarproof doesn't mean that you remove all sugar from your home and prevent your kids from enjoying treats. It *does* mean that you, as a parent, recognize that your children can't avoid the sugar storm. It means that you use strategies that are designed to bring your kids' sugar consumption down to a reasonable level—and that you teach your children how to protect themselves and make good choices.

Making your kids Sugarproof will involve activities that help your children recognize the sources and dangers of high sugar intake and take action to reduce and minimize consumption. It's our way to protect kids from the overly sweet environment that they have to navigate every single day. This part of the book suggests several activities to get you started, along with tools and techniques to ensure their success. In the next chapter, we'll show you seven strategies designed to Sugarproof your children and your family; you can choose the ones that seem best for your family, or you can tackle them all. And if you're the type of parent who appreciates a structured program, you can try either or both of the two plans that follow: the 7-Day No-Added-Sugar Challenge or the 28-Day Challenge: A Gradual Plan for Rightsizing Sugar. Either plan will help you identify the sources of excess sugars in your family and then rightsize your family's intake. You can choose the one that seems better suited to the way your children respond to change, or you can try both. No matter which plan you use, you'll modify the way your family consumes sugar. And from this healthy home base, you can then equip your children with the tools for moderating sugar intake when they are out in the world. They'll develop self-regulation, a skill they can use for life.

Our techniques have been tested on real families, and they're designed to be easy for both parents and kids. They'll be even easier if you do some prep work ahead of time, and that's what we'll cover now. This preparation involves communication, getting everyone motivated to change, creating a low-sugar home environment, and anticipating tricky scenarios.

We like to begin with communication. Long-term, the Sugarproof approach won't work if you simply tell your children what they can and can't eat. Forcing kids to do anything, from homework to taking out the garbage, can result in grumbling and complaints, and creating an over-restrictive food culture at home will backfire. Ordering them to give up sugar completely "because it's bad for you" isn't going to be successful.

Michael's daughter saw this effect firsthand. Her school allows the class to visit local shops for lunch break. On the Monday after Easter, one of her friends bought a bag of chocolate candy for lunch and ate the whole thing in one sitting. Michael's daughter asked why she would eat so much candy all at once. Her friend explained that her family's Easter gathering at a relative's house didn't involve any candy or sweets. Instead the Easter bunny brought celery and boiled eggs. Her friend felt deprived and struck back.

Yes, our kids live in a sugar storm. But resist the belief that you can protect your kids by creating an overly restrictive environment. Instead, have a series of family conversations, ones that go both ways. You get to have a say—and so do your kids. A strategic family dialogue will help get everyone motivated and on board.

What is the fine line between finding a way to cut back on sugar and turning into the sugar police? How do you begin the conversation? How do you start to change your child's relationship with sugar without destroying special holidays, birthday parties, visits with grandparents, or hangout time with friends? We've got some tested tips for you. We'll walk you through the process and ultimately help you involve your children in their own success.

I Did It My Way: The Magic of Internal Motivation

The goal of *Sugarproof* is to reduce sugar without creating a restrictive environment. In order to teach kids how to make changes on their own terms, you can learn to promote what health professionals call *internal or intrinsic motivation*. When people are driven by internal motivation, they are more likely to make positive health decisions on a consistent basis. You can harness its principles at home and inspire your kids to adopt healthier eating behaviors on their own terms. Children who act with internal motivation feel like they're making their own choices. We often hear kids say that they're driven to cut down sugar because they want to fit better in their clothes, or they want to stay more focused in class, or they want to have clearer skin. Your children will have their own motives for cutting down sugar—and that's the key. Their motives have to be their own, not yours or ours or some other kid's.

Contrast internal motivation with motivation that comes from the outside. External motivation involves engaging in a behavior for a reward such as money, approval, or extra hours of screen time. You might motivate your kids to eat less candy over spring break in exchange for an increase in allowance or time watching Netflix, but they won't develop their own reasons for choosing to have less candy in the future. You'll be stuck having to reward your children each time you try to get them to reduce or avoid sugar.

You can help your children explore and develop their own reasons and internal motivations for making healthy changes to their diet—and ultimately learn the ability to self-regulate without the need for an external reward. Psychology research has found that we all have three basic needs that, if met, will make us want to act in ways that promote our health. These three basic needs are competence, relatedness, and autonomy. When you engage kids with these needs in mind, you make it easier for them to succeed.

Competence

Competence is our desire for a sense of mastery. Boost your children's sense of competence by teaching them about what's good for their bodies—and empower them to help make snacks and meals. With some knowledge and skills, even the youngest of kids can start to understand how to make healthier eating choices:

- Children aren't usually concerned about their future health, so it helps to connect their sugar consumption to things they do care about, such as being strong and athletic, doing well on exams, being able to pay attention for a whole movie, or having better skin.

- Depending on their age, you could talk to your children about what happens to food after it's eaten and the ways in which the nutrients in food are used by the body.

- Ask questions that help your kids become more aware about how their bodies respond to sugar. Do they have more energy, can they think more clearly on mornings when they haven't had a sugary breakfast? Did they feel tired and worn out after they had a soda with friends?

- Explain to kids how the food industry works. Engage in conversations about our overly sweet food supply and how the food industry manipulates kids through advertising and social media gimmicks. Jessica, one of the moms participating in our 7-Day Challenge, said she was able to "open up powerful conversations" with her children on this topic. She told them, "There are some people whose job is to see what is the perfect combination of fat, sugar, and salt to make our brains keep wanting more and more and more. There is a reason why you want to keep going back for those McDonald's pancakes." Teaching kids that they are being manipulated into making poor choices about food is eye-opening for them. After their conversation, Jessica's seven-year-old son started pointing out examples of advertising.

- Teach your kids how to read ingredient lists and spot added sugar and sweeteners. Once they learn how to spot added sugar, they'll discover that sugar is *everywhere.*

- Take kids to the grocery store. Taking young children with you can be a challenge, but for kids of all ages, it's a chance to learn about food. Let them help select new fruits and vegetables or other products they like but with less sugar. Food shopping helps build independent skills.

- Involve kids in cooking. It can help you save time and increases their willingness to eat less sweet options. We realize that when you are busy or stressed, it can seem like more work to get young children involved. Prepping dinner alone can give you a moment of peace and make less of a mess. But there are enough other benefits from involving kids in food prep that it's worth making time to do it when possible. See Part 3 for ideas on how to involve kids of various ages and actually lighten your own workload. Food prep time together also gives you an opportunity to open up a conversation around sugar, diet, and health in a more relaxed environment. As kids get older and become preteens or teens, they can even be responsible for an entire simple meal.

Relatedness

Relatedness, in the context of food, means how we use food to connect to others. This area can be difficult for children, especially teenagers, to master. For example, teens often focus on what might be perceived as cool or not cool. Food is such a large and important part of the social fabric for kids that it can drive poor choices like choosing a fast-food lunch to be with school friends over the healthy packed lunch they brought to eat that day, or getting a soda at the movies because everyone else is getting one.

It's not just social situations with friends that can be tricky. Family dynamics can become an obstacle to healthy eating. Kids are notorious for making a fuss about what is served or getting bored quickly at the table, and parent–child power struggles can prevent kids from making healthy choices. Additionally, many family gatherings revolve around sharing meals, and family members often provide sweets as a means of showing love.

Here are some ideas for helping your children navigate the social aspects of food:

- When friends come over, invite them to participate in activities such as the sweet spot experiment (page 251) or the Clif Bar Challenge (page 50). And offer them healthy options for snacks. Once you get out of the sugary snack rut, you will find quite a few options out there that taste great and that your children and their friends will enjoy, especially if they can be involved in preparing them. You can even send extras to school in your child's lunch for sharing.

- Make Sugarproof snacks, dishes, and treats for social gatherings. You'll be surprised at how many adults will thank you for supplying something healthy.

- Get the entire family involved. Of course, every family is different. Some parents and siblings may be more willing than others to join in making major diet changes. Don't worry if you can't get everyone in the family on board right away. It might be a gradual process that will take time. Point out the overall health benefits that everyone can see and try to build excitement around any successes that you experience.

- Plan meals for the week, and do it with input from the entire family. When your kids have a say in meal planning, they'll be more excited about eating—even when they're eating lower-sugar options. Pick a time when everyone is together to brainstorm a list of favorite meals or identify new recipes to try. If you have more than one child, let each choose a breakfast or weeknight dinner that is in harmony with your goals. Other benefits of a meal plan: You won't feel like a short-order cook, making different meals for each person in the family, and you won't have to default to convenience foods, takeout, or going to a restaurant, where you have less control over what is in the food.

- Try to avoid allowing kids to eat in front of the television, iPad, or other device. This promotes mindless eating, whereas sitting down together for a "family meal," even if it is just two family members together, helps improve the quality of what kids eat.

Autonomy

When you give your kids the ability to make educated decisions, you're building their autonomy, the longing to control the course of one's own life. Ultimately, your children will be the ones making decisions out in the world, from what to order at Starbucks with friends to how much candy to eat on a school trip. Here are some suggestions to help build autonomy in the context of food:

- Ease up and relax. It's hard as a parent or caregiver to trust your children will make the right decision about sugar, but if you give them some space, they can make their own decisions in their own time. Let them decide what treat they want on a given day or what dish they might learn to prepare next. Older kids might want to research and discover their own snacks or new items to try. Let them come to you with options and learn about them together.

- Let them be the boss. Say you're at a buffet and there is a large selection of desserts. Your children want them all. Ask them what they think would be a reasonable amount of dessert and see if you can use that as a starting point in a discussion.

- Be a good example and role model. Let them see you following the same guidelines they are for regulating and moderating sugar. Together you can practice, internalize, and change.

- Let your children make their own mistakes. Trust your children to navigate situations out of the house on their own without policing and micromanaging. If you do talk to them about their choices, try to refrain from being overly critical. They won't always get it right, but you can guide them and they'll learn from their mistakes and work toward autonomy sooner if they know they're making their own decisions. When they do eat or drink too much sugar, help them evaluate the results in how their body feels. Did it cause a stomachache or make them tired or grouchy?

Communicate Motivational Change with RULE

Instead of announcing your intent to reduce sugar and then expecting your kids to follow along, get your kids involved from the start and customize your strategies together. The extent of their involvement will depend on their ages, but you can include even preschool-age children in the process. As you begin a conversation about sugar and your desire to try a new way of eating, help your children explore their worries as well as reasons they might be in favor of change. We use this strategy, known as motivational interviewing, in our clinical studies. Because it's specifically designed to promote internal motivation for changing health behaviors, it helps kids start off on the right foot. You can also use it to help your kids select what they are willing to work on, which increases their active participation.

Practitioners of motivational interviewing go through rigorous training before they use it in a clinical setting, but its basic principles are easy to learn. With a little thought and practice, you can begin to incorporate these principles into any family discussion you have about sugar. The technique involves asking open questions, active listening, and providing useful information. There are four guiding principles you can use for putting the theory behind motivational change into successful action, known by the acronym RULE:

R = Roll with resistance
U = Understand your child's own motivation
L = Listen with empathy
E = Empower your child

You can use these principles as you see fit, and not necessarily in this order. They'll help you establish two-way communication and prepare for any negative reactions. It's too much to expect that your children will become excited at the thought of reducing sugar, but if you keep using the RULE guidelines, you'll find that their resistance will soften and that they will warm to the idea of change.

Roll with resistance.

The thought of making changes to eating habits can feel threatening to kids. (Adults, too.) Older children may feel judged, and younger ones may just simply not want to give up their favorite sweet treats. What do you do? You roll with resistance. Try to be empathetic instead of attempting to persuade them. Talk about whatever they bring up. Instead of attempting to persuade them that you're right and they're wrong, hear what specifically worries them and why. Lunch at school? Saturday afternoons out with friends? Football practice? As you listen, remind yourself what it felt like to be a kid. Not getting to enjoy certain treats can mean something different to them than it does to you.

Your kids might be unwilling to talk about the subject entirely. If they've pushed back, next time ask their permission to start the talk: "Would you mind if we talked a little about how we eat as a family?" Try bringing up the conversation at a time when your child is not overly hungry, stressed, or tired. In addition, make sure you yourself are feeling patient, open, and tolerant before you start the conversation. Don't do it when you are short on time or energy. Be gentle, kind, and understanding so they know they're not in trouble or that you're not mad at them if things don't work out. We like to frame the Sugarproof process as an experiment that can be fun, rather than as a set of rules that need to be enforced. It can be helpful to broach the topic by suggesting a fun activity, like going to the farmer's market together to buy some fruits and vegetables, or heading to the grocery store together specifically to look for foods or snacks that are low in sugar. Sometimes conversations come more easily while you are engaged in an activity rather than when you are sitting down face-to-face. Framing is also important. Kids can't always perceive health risks. If they can't relate to issues that seem abstract, then you can say something like: "As your parent, I care about you and want to help you learn how to keep your body healthy."

Understand your child's own motivation.

You are trying to help lead your children toward healthier behavior, and for this to work, they need to feel personally accepted and valued. So instead of listing reasons why your child should eat less sugar, guide them toward their *own* reasons for eating in a healthier way. Try questions like "How do you think you might benefit if you have less sugar?" or "What will happen if you don't make any changes?" or "How much sugar do you think you need"? If they are having trouble coming up with ideas, you could mention some reasons why other people decide to try eating less sugar and how they go about it. One effective strategy is to emphasize that any changes are time limited, while leaving future changes as possibilities. For example, you could say, "This is just a change in what we are going to eat this week, and then we can see how we feel and decide what to do after that."

Listen with empathy.

Listening with empathy will also help you understand your child's concerns and help your children *know* that you are hearing them. Ask them how they feel about cutting back on sugar. If you work toward a solution together, they will know you are on their side and both of you are invested. For example, if your child is grumbling about having to give up their favorite breakfast cereal, plan a trip to the store together to find a new one. Or if they are not happy about giving up ice cream during the 7-Day Challenge, let them know that they can have other alternatives like Whole Fruit Pops (see page 330).

Empower your child.

Acting as the sugar police won't improve your child's health or their internal motivation. It's better that you empower your children. As you talk things through, let them know that they can make choices. They can help create a meal plan and include their favorites for dinner. At the coffee shop, ask them what they would choose from the menu and help them troubleshoot how to lower the sugar content or compare sugar amounts in the different drinks. As you'll see when you learn about the 7-Day and 28-Day Challenges, you can also make a menu of options or prioritize a list of health goals to try. From there, your children can help select some first steps.

As you use the RULE principles to communicate with your kids, you might hear thoughts and feelings that are different than you expected. If you have multiple children, their responses may vary dramatically. As you'll see, the 7-Day and 28-Day Challenges give you the flexibility to respond to their motivations, concerns, and suggestions. You might be hoping to make changes to your seven-year-old's lunch, but he or she says they'll feel uncomfortable with their friends. Maybe together you decide to start with changes at home; you can revisit the topic of school lunches or snacks later. Your teen might feel overwhelmed and not sure where to start. Make a menu of options or prioritize a list of health goals to try. From there, your teen can help select some first steps.

The Readiness Ruler

If your children are unsure if they want to make any changes, you can use an approach called the *readiness ruler*. To do this, ask your child "on a scale of 1 to 5, how willing are you to make the change?" If they are not very willing (low on the scale, say a 1 or 2), then you can ask if there is anything that might make them more willing. This gives you a chance to explore what your children's barriers are toward making the change.

Another useful strategy is to activate the *upstander* in your kids, the part of them that wants to make their own decisions and not be tricked into things. Talk to them about aggressive and confusing marketing tactics used by the food industry that specifically target kids and that encourage them to consume more sugar. Tell them how much sugar is considered safe or healthy for growing kids relative to the sugar content of specific products marketed toward kids. Not only does this strategy help kids develop critical thinking skills, it also helps shift the focus to food industry practices rather than "my strict family."

The more your kids are involved in the plan, the more willing they will be to participate. Remember Grace from Chapter 4, who was falling asleep in class? She realized that a lower-sugar breakfast was helping her stay awake and keep her focus. This inspired her to also choose Sugarproof after-school snacks like apple slices with almond butter, and she learned that doing this helped her finish her homework faster so she could spend more time with her friends. She developed the internal motivation to make some beneficial changes.

As Grace's experience shows, the physical and mental benefits of reducing sugar can be significant. We confidently predict that you and your family will notice these changes. So perhaps the easiest strategy is to ask your kids to try our plans. Once kids start noticing that they feel better with less sugar, they will need less convincing from you about the dangers of too much sugar.

Create a Healthy Refuge

After communication, the next way to lay the groundwork for Sugarproof success is to create a healthy, low-sugar home environment. Either strategy alone won't work nearly as well as the combination. Joy, a mom from Portland, discovered the power of a positive home environment when she and her family did our 7-Day Challenge. As part of the process, she and her husband Sugarproofed their home, and they were surprised by how well it went over. After she completed the plan and thought about how she wanted to move forward, she noted, "My kids get enough sugar outside of the house, so that can be their sugar for the week." In other words, even after the challenge, Joy and her husband decided they wanted to maintain a low-sugar environment in their home.

Your home should be a safe refuge where kids won't have to navigate around constant sugary obstacles, like they do almost everywhere else. If there are sodas in the refrigerator, cookies in the cupboard, and ice cream in the freezer, someone is going to end up eating them. The easiest way to start is to eliminate as many temptations as possible. How rigorous you want to be is up to you and your family. (If you sense that your family is going to have a tough time giving up their treats, you might want to try the 28-Day Challenge, which is designed to give you a slower, more gradual entry into the Sugarproof process and doesn't ask you to get rid of sugary temptations right away.)

If you shift the focus from what you *don't* want in your home to what you *do* want, you might find you can displace the bad foods simply by providing a strong selection of healthier alternatives. Your kids won't miss the cookies as much if they find homemade energy bites (page 319) already made and waiting. They won't feel as deprived of soda if there is sparkling water with fresh lime in your fridge. They might be fine with less sugary breakfast cereals if there is a nice bowl of berries or cut fruit available at breakfast time to top low-sugar cereals.

As you're working to improve your home food environment, think about what is sitting out on the kitchen counter. A sugar bowl or cookie jar? A box of hot chocolate mix? Sugary breakfast cereal? Seeing pre-made snacks or convenience foods prompts kids to think about consuming them. But if your children walk into the kitchen and see a bowl of fruit or jar of nuts on the counter, they will be more likely to have a healthy snack. Moving sugary things out of plain view can have a big impact on eating habits with minimal effort. If you keep the honey or sugar out on the counter near the oatmeal or tea, using it becomes a habit by association, but if it is stored in an upper cabinet, it will be less likely to be used.

There can be a few other benefits—and challenges, too—to making your home a safe zone. Tabatha, a mom from Seattle who participated in our 7-Day Challenge, told us she often found herself on autopilot in the grocery store, buying sweets aimlessly. She noticed herself thinking: "I should just make sure we have a carton of ice cream." As Tabatha explained, "In my brain I had this checklist of stuff I should have in my house. This challenge made me pause." In the grocery store one day, she was about to buy some sweets when she thought to herself, "I don't need this."

As Tabatha pointed out, "A by-product of buying less sugar is that you save money."

You may spend more on fresh fruits and vegetables, but you will save by not buying as many convenience or processed products. Make a list for the grocery store and stick to it. Additionally, make sure you have the ingredients on hand to support your new breakfast and lunch plans; otherwise, it is easy to slip back into old habits. Joy found that with some planning, she could easily solve snack problems by making some of the Sugarproof recipes like the Sugarproof Granola and Granola Thins (page 295). She reported back: "The boys love the granola. Daniel says it doesn't really taste like a sugary treat, but he loves it. Lucas told me to put it in his snack and his lunch for school tomorrow. Yes! This is easy!"

Planning your weekly meals in advance is a key to success if you're a parent or caregiver with limited time for cooking. Between work, school, extracurricular activities, and errands, most parents need to be extra efficient with their time in the kitchen. Here are some ideas to help ensure your home remains a healthy, Sugarproof environment:

1. **Stock a Sugarproof pantry.** Use the Sugarproof staples shopping list in Part 3, "The Sugarproof Kitchen: Recipes and Tips," to help you determine what you'll need to keep on hand. These staples can form the basis for a variety of snacks and meals. Although it's best to buy fresh and/or unprocessed foods, it's fine if you'd like to buy a few convenience foods to keep on hand in case you need a quick meal. Just check the ingredient lists carefully to make sure they have little to no sugar or no low-calorie sweeteners.

2. **Keep track of your successes.** Jot down a list of your family's most popular and successful menu ideas, categorized by meal. Use this list to plan for the week and talk to everyone to get their input on breakfast, lunch, and dinner. You will likely run into differences of opinion, and that's okay. Along the way, you'll learn some new things from your children that should help prevent frustrating scenarios of spending time cooking—only to find out they've decided they don't like that dish anymore. You'll begin to hear clearer answers: "Mom, I like your chili, but not when it has chunks of onion in it."

3. **Find new options for packed lunches.** Families often struggle to come up with new options to replace granola bars and other lunch items. It's perfectly fine if you don't have time to make an entire packed lunch from scratch. Good convenience snacks include cheese, nuts, seeds, edamame, seaweed snacks, carrots, trail mix (with no candy or added sugar), or cups of plain yogurt with fresh fruit. Our 7-day and 28-day plans include even more ideas for options.

Containers Matter

When it comes to school lunch, keeping your child's favorite foods and snacks accessible, temperature controlled, and easy to manage can make the difference between what gets eaten and what doesn't. As Samantha, a mom who completed our 28-Day Challenge, explained, "It seems to be all about the container for my kids. When they get the containers that they like, they eat pretty much anything in there." She's right. Kids respond to lunches that are packed well, with containers that they find attractive and that are sized to fit their portions.

For a successful lunch, your kids will need a good insulated lunch box or tote. And you'll need a supply of large and small containers, along with freezer packs, on hand. Get a good insulated Thermos for soup and other hot foods. Stainless steel containers can help separate different items, are rugged, and can last for years. They also limit exposure to plastic. Keep trying until you find what works for you and your kids' healthy eating plan.

Batch cook.

Prepping ingredients, side dishes, or entrées in batches will save you time. It also limits food waste and makes a huge difference in the quality of family meals. The best items to cook ahead are vegetables because they can then be used in so many ways. You can make the Roasted Vegetable Master Recipe (page 312) on a Sunday like Jessica did, using sweet potatoes, butternut squash, red peppers, and kale. Add them to a veggie wrap, then a burrito bowl, and even into soup. As Jessica said happily, the kids "were all over it." So was her husband, Matteo. Or try the Roasted Red Cabbage Crisps (page 314). It's simple, inexpensive, easy, and a game changer in terms of getting everyone to enjoy vegetables.

Freeze strategically.

Many of the items you make in batches can also be frozen and used in subsequent weeks. You don't have to have the same soup two nights in a row if you freeze the leftovers. Plus, having a freezer meal or two available is so useful when you have had an extra-long day and just don't have time to cook. It's also a great way to take advantage of the seasonal availability of favorite fruits and vegetables or of sales that let you save by buying in bulk. Our Sugarproof treats and muffins can also be frozen. You may not have time to make Easy No-Bake Energy Bites (page 319) or No-Bake Chocolate Sesame Squares (page 328) every week, but you might be able to find fifteen minutes once a month to make a double or even triple batch. Then freeze them so you can pull them out as needed for lunch box treats or after-school snacks.

Try a Farm Share or CSA

For fresh-from-the-garden fruits and vegetables, consider a farm share. Most communities have Community Supported Agriculture (CSA) programs that allow you to go in with other families to support a farmer or gardener in exchange for a box of fresh veggies and fruit every week. The bounty, often including kale, lettuce, squash, strawberries, peaches, asparagus, broccoli, cabbage, cucumbers, okra, herbs, and more, can be plentiful and a delicious way to teach kids about seasonal eating. It also changes up your veggie routine. CSA fruits and vegetables are local and usually organic. They're also a cost-effective way to ensure you always have fresh produce in the house. You and your kids will enjoy opening the box to see what's inside every week. A quick online search should reveal options in your area.

Prep fruit and raw vegetables.

We suggest washing, cutting, and chopping fruit and raw vegetables and keeping them handy in the refrigerator for breakfasts, lunches, and snacks. If possible, use clear glass containers for storage so everyone can see what's in them (of course, this is also better than plastic for the environment). It's easy for your kids to eat well if they can open the refrigerator and grab melon cubes or carrot sticks, whereas finding a whole melon or unpeeled carrots can be an obstacle, especially for small children. Keeping cut-up lemon and lime wedges in the refrigerator is also a great way to make still or sparkling water more interesting for anyone who wants the cold bubbles of soda without the sugar.

Celebrations

Dessert is a centerpiece of most celebrations. Birthdays, holidays, school functions, and even family parties often have cakes, cookies, candy, or other sweets as a focal point. Sometimes there is not only a cake toward the end of a party but also a table full of sweets to snack on throughout the party as well. It's enough to throw a wrench into almost any of your attempts to reduce sugar. But it's possible to enjoy celebrations while keeping the sugar at a moderate level. The key is to find a strategy that you can use routinely as a party guest—or even a party host. Here are some ideas for different situations.

Hosting parties

If you are hosting a party, especially a kids' party, try offering the kids a wholesome snack or a light meal early in the event. Ideally this would not include sweets at all, but some type of protein as well as fiber from whole grains, vegetables, and maybe some fruit. You might try starting with assorted small sandwiches on whole-grain bread, pizza with a whole-grain crust and a few vegetables as toppings, or snack platters of hummus, olives, deli meats, cheeses, veggies with dip, or chopped fruit. If the kids can fill up at the party on better options, it will keep their appetites more satisfied and reduce the frenzy over the cake. Try not to create one of those buffets of sweet foods and drinks where the kids can serve themselves. If you have a piñata or make goody bags, mix in alternative prizes like stickers, small toys, or craft supplies.

Attending parties

If you know your children are attending a party where there's likely to be a large number of sweets, try serving a well balanced meal beforehand. Encourage your children to choose water at the party as a beverage instead of sweet drinks, which frees up space in the sugar budget for cake or dessert. If there is a large number of treats to choose from, encourage kids to pick one that they most want to enjoy. Often there are kids at parties following a specific diet such as gluten-free or vegan, so encourage your child to ask if there is also an option that is lower in sugar and doesn't contain low-calorie sweeteners.

Slumber parties can be a challenge because they can involve multiple meals and snacks. Tabatha's children were going to so many slumber parties that it was getting in the way of their Sugarproof efforts. Between the celebratory cake or cupcakes, all the candy the kids like to snack on through the night, and the usual pancakes and syrup for breakfast the next day, it was just too much. As a new approach, Tabatha began not only to feed her daughters a solid meal before going to the party but also talked with the host parents about how her family was taking steps to reduce sugar and sent her kids with a few healthy, low-sugar snacks. One mom even offered Tabatha's daughter a no added-sugar version of the pancakes she made for breakfast.

Other holidays

Beyond birthdays, we all have to navigate the specific "candy" holidays like Halloween, Valentine's Day, and Easter. Finding the right balance between cutting sugar completely and making the holiday a special celebration is a challenge that will require conversations. It's not that uncommon for parents to assign more meaning to special treats than kids who may be just as happy with limited sweets along with alternative, nonfood "treats." When the candy holidays come around, ask your kids what they'd rather have and think creatively about how to minimize the sugar load. For Valentine's Day and Easter, use nonfood gifts to celebrate (like flowers, books, gift cards, or certificates for special time with Mom or Dad). For Halloween, try "The Switch Witch," which involves having your kids leave a large portion of candy that they collected out for a witch who comes overnight and switches it for a small gift or money. Also, if you end up on sugar overload after any of these celebrations, you can always reset your household with the 7-Day No-Added-Sugar Challenge.

Holiday Gifts

Instead of grabbing prepackaged candy or making cookies, give teachers and others non-sweet gifts. Teachers suffer from sugar overload, too, and they are often deeply grateful for alternatives like gift certificates to restaurants or coffee shops they like, books, handmade crafts, flowers or plants, special tea, or a scented candle.

When Your Kids Eat Their Feelings

Eating is often about issues beyond satisfying hunger. Sometimes, emotions prompt us to eat even when we don't feel hungry. This phenomenon, called *eating in the absence of hunger*, is well documented in children but of course is not unique to them. Eating for reasons other than being hungry can happen when we are happy, celebrating, bored, stressed, or sad. Before you start to reduce sugar in your family's diet, think about possible emotional connections with sugar. Here are a few common scenarios, along with some strategies for managing them.

Stress and sugar

Many of us gravitate to sugar in times of stress. Sometimes that stress is sudden and acute. All families go through tragedies, from the death of a close family member to job loss or divorce. During these times, neighbors, extended family, and friends often help with much-appreciated meals and gifts of food. And who hasn't had a stressful day that ended with a container of ice cream? Eating when we're under acute stress makes us feel better, thanks to dopamine. During a rough emotional patch, you might shift away from healthy eating habits, which only makes an already stressful situation worse. Think about the steps you can take to get back to normal. It might seem like extra sweets help you or your kids get through trying times, like a major move, birth, or travel, but the opposite is true. Eating less sugar will ultimately help reduce stress. If you find that your kids are moody, irritable, or not sleeping during these phases, remember that sugar could be adding to the problems.

While acute stress can be incredibly disruptive, chronic stress can be even more damaging to the family's eating habits. Chronic illness, financial strain, overly busy schedules, or even a parent's relationship worries may leave the entire family too stressed and busy to eat well. Prolonged periods of chronic stress can cause healthy eating habits to go by the wayside for months or years on end.

Often we parents struggle to model healthy eating when we are under chronic stress. Candice, one of the moms we worked with, posted a picture on Instagram of a ziplock bag that contained packages of Sour Patch gummies and caramel popcorn. It was labeled with the date and said, "Belongs to Mom!" Her post said, "Do not touch my snacks! These are my emergency stress relievers. I'll know you did so don't try me!" It was a funny post—but Candice was unintentionally sending her kids the clear message that sugar is a stress reliever. Nathan, a dad who participated in our 7-Day Challenge along with his family, discovered that he needed to address his habit of stress-eating in the evenings. Of all his family members, it was Nathan who had the hardest time with the challenge. Under stress at work, he helped put the kids to bed but then came back downstairs to make himself chocolate milk or to rummage around in the cabinets for sweet snacks.

Though difficult, it is possible to retrain yourself to find other ways to manage stress that don't involve sugar. Jessica experienced a turnaround with stress-related sugar cravings during the 7-Day Challenge. As she explained, "I have a major sweet tooth. I started drinking coffee recently because I was so stressed. It was the Nestlé Coffee-mate French Vanilla Creamer that I was craving—the sweetness, not the caffeine." After completing the challenge, Jessica gave us the following update: "Now I'm no longer having coffee in the morning. As a result, I started going to bed earlier and my sleep habits improved."

The problem is that when parents stress-eat—or comfort themselves with food—children adopt the same behavior. They can see parents using sweets as an emotional crutch and form their own stress-eating habit. Before you begin to Sugarproof your children, think of your own relationship with sugar. If you are an emotional eater who turns to food, specifically sweets, for comfort, then you may want to seek other outlets for emotions like taking a walk, talking with a friend, having a bath, or any other activity that helps relieve stress.

Consoling sadness with sugar

It's tempting to use sugar as a quick fix for cheering up our kids, or ourselves. But there's a fine line between the occasional treat and using sugar as a crutch for sadness. Kids have big emotions, which can sometimes overwhelm parents. When we know that giving children something sweet works quickly to restore a happy mood or distract from impending tears, it can be easy to use this tactic again and again. But be careful. Some little kids realize that if they cry, they will be consoled with sweets, so they continue crying, hoping for the same "reward." Instead of consoling your children with sugar, trying consoling them with a hug, a back rub, or a relaxing activity like taking a walk, reading, or watching a movie together.

Showing love

Joy said, "My dad's love language is providing sweets for the family." He was affectionately known for bringing ice cream and pies and cakes to Joy and her siblings and all of the grandkids. And he loved seeing how his homemade chocolate chip pancakes made everyone happy. Plus, these gestures increased his popularity with the grandkids, which added to his own happiness. When Joy started working on our 7-Day Challenge, she decided to talk with her dad about limiting sweets with her children to smaller portions served less frequently, and he was willing to oblige. He started offering fresh berries with his pancakes instead of mixing chocolate chips into them.

You may decide to ask certain friends or family members not to buy your children sweets. I (Emily) have a family friend who was in the habit of bringing cookies or candy each time she came to visit. It was her way of showing love. But the sweets were piling up from all the visits. I decided to ask her gently if she could skip bringing sweets for the boys. She didn't mind at all and instead began to bring homemade Thai food.

Sometimes grandparents and other family members and friends are willing to provide alternate treats and snacks, but they are just not sure what these other options could be. You can help by giving them ideas. One mom who participated in our 7-Day Challenge even gave her parents a list of foods to have in the house before she brought the kids for a visit. Substitutions like Cheerios instead of Cinnamon Toast Crunch or regular crackers instead of graham crackers can make a big difference when you're trying to cut sugar. Her parents were happy to oblige, and her kids were happy with the available options at Grandma and Grandpa's house.

Sugar as a bribe or reward

It can be so easy to reward or even bribe your kids with sugar, because it usually works. The problem is the slippery slope that bribery creates. If you reward your children with sweets for a good grade on a test, soon kids expect treats for *every* good grade, or for making their beds, or taking out the trash. As you consider alternatives, try offering rewards of doing fun things together, such as reading a book after dinner or going outside and practicing soccer. Using sugar as a reward can derail your work of reducing sugar, so look for other reward strategies like a new book from the bookstore, new craft supplies, a family bike ride, or any other activity that your child wants to do.

Tricky Scenarios

Now comes the tough part. You have the tools for the conversations, and some prompts to keep kids engaged—but you're a parent, and you know that life doesn't always go according to a plan in a book. Don't worry. You can anticipate some of the bumps in the road. Several of the families we've worked with have posed their tricky scenarios to us, and together we've come up with solutions that you can also use when needed.

"How can I prevent outbursts at the grocery store?"

As she began to reduce sugar with her two-year-old son, Rachel was concerned that she wouldn't be able to manage his emotional outbursts in the grocery store. When she took him shopping, she usually bought sweetened rice cakes to snack on at the store. Now that she knew how many added sugars are in these treats, she wasn't sure what to do when he asked for them in the grocery store. If she said "no," he started screaming.

Rachel's solution

Rachel continued to say "no" to the rice cakes—but she also found replacement items that didn't have added sugars, like cheese, cashews, dried unsweetened fruit, savory popcorn, or seaweed snacks. Or she would simply buy plain rice crackers. Offering options kept him interested, and he enjoyed that he could still pick out a special treat while in the store.

"My child never eats anything. Will he starve?"

Catherine, one of the moms who did our 7-Day Challenge, told us that she was concerned that her six-year-old son Zack was too skinny. "He has eating days and non-eating days. When it's a non-eating day, I'm so glad that he's willing to ingest anything that I give him what he wants just to get some nutrition into him. Not ice cream for breakfast—but if he wants waffles and juice, I'll give it to him. Zack used to eat so many foods. Now he won't even eat chicken nuggets. What should I do?"

Catherine's solution

Giving Zack sweets just to get him to eat *something* was aggravating the situation. It lowered the chances that he would eat healthier options. Instead, Catherine began to put a variety of healthy foods on the table at breakfast, such as a bowl of blueberries, low-sugar cereal, whole-grain toast with peanut butter, scrambled eggs, or our Sugarproof muffins (Blueberry Banana Muffins, page 288), and let Zack choose. If he decided not to eat, that was okay, too. She started to give less attention to Zack at meals. Sometimes picky eating can be a power struggle, and Catherine realized that if she just left him alone and didn't force him, Zack would eventually eat. Maybe not at the current meal, but perhaps at the next one. Either way, he wasn't going to starve.

"But my friend gets to eat it. Why can't I?"

Annie's six-year-old asked for a Nutella sandwich in her lunch because her best friend Isabelle got one every day. When Annie said no, her daughter told her that it wasn't fair, and that Isabelle's mom was nicer than she was.

Annie's solution

Annie bought a small jar of Nutella and allowed her daughter to have this treat on occasion but not as a regular lunch staple. She talked with her daughter and explained that for their family, this sandwich fell into the treat category. Her daughter could choose to have it, but she knew it was her treat for that day.

"My kid is spending his allowance on sugar!"

Jo realized that her twelve-year-old, Eli, was using his allowance money to buy candy and soda every day on the way home from school with his friends.

Jo's solution

During a relaxed moment, Jo decided to talk with Eli and tell him gently that she knows he likes to stop for snacks with his friends, but she was concerned that if he went every day, it could add up to a lot of sugar. She mentioned that she was most concerned about the soda, and asked if he would be willing to have sparkling water or if she could buy him a new water bottle to bring with him. They also talked about swapping the candy for trail mix or nuts or dried fruit at least on some days. Finally, she asked Eli if there was anything she could buy or make to put in his backpack for after school that would help him not to buy things at the store, and he said that he really liked the No-Bake Chocolate Sesame Squares (page 328). Eli can even make them for himself, so after their talk they went to the store to buy the ingredients.

"I'm alone in this! Why can't you support me?"

Renee told her ex-husband that she wanted their kids to eat less sugar. However, he continued to take them to the movies and buy them candy, soda, and ice cream and then told them not to tell their mom about it. How can Renee talk to her co-parenting spouse without putting him on the defensive, even though she feels betrayed? And does she need to give up on trying to Sugarproof?

Renee's solution

After a few failed attempts to get her ex-husband on board, Renee decided to drop the issue with him. Meanwhile, she began to focus on things she had more control over, like what she would buy at the grocery store for everyday staples for her house. She also worked with her children to teach them some of the Sugarproof principles so that they could start making healthier choices on their own. Eventually they no longer wanted a soda at the movies when they went with their dad. Renee was able to drop her perceived role as the "bad guy," and her ex-husband began to notice that the kids seemed better behaved with less sugar, which in turn convinced him that moderating sugar was indeed worthwhile.

Eyes on the Prize: Self-Regulation

Ultimately, the goal of the Sugarproof approach is to help children develop independent decision-making skills. Parents can't be around all the time, so kids need to know how to choose wisely and how to tell when they've had enough. Eventually, they'll grow up to be adults who can eat sugar in moderation—and who don't suffer the effects of diabetes, heart disease, or other conditions that can be brought on by chronic, excess sugar consumption.

Starting a conversation with your children about sugar helps bring them into the process. If you combine these conversations with a low-sugar home environment, then you can provide a healthy foundation for your child to grow into a young adult who makes wise, independent decisions. It is even easier for kids to learn about good choices when their parents use some tried-and-true strategies to reduce sugar. In the next chapter, we'll show you how to master them.

To view the scientific references cited in this chapter, please visit us online at sugarproofkids.com/bibliography.

CHAPTER SEVEN

Cutting Sugar: Seven Sugarproof Strategies That Work

Now it's time to talk about some specific strategies for change. We have found that seven simple strategies are key to the success of Sugarproof. Supported with research, these strategies work for kids and adults. They're even more effective when the entire family implements them together. How many you tackle at once is up to you. Some families like to start with one or two strategies that seem the most doable, and build from that; others implement all of them at the same time.

SEVEN SUGARPROOF STRATEGIES:

1. Set everyone up for success with breakfast.
2. Ditch the liquid sugar.
3. Avoid fructose.
4. Use snacks to your advantage.
5. Choose sweet treats wisely.
6. Set guidelines for major culprits.
7. Work a menu like a pro.

Sugarproof Strategy #1: Set Everyone up for Success with Breakfast

Dr. Jekyll or Mr. Hyde? Some kids can be either, depending on what they eat in the morning. When breakfast lacks protein but is full of sugar—think toast with jam or a pastry—most kids will take a ride on the sugar roller coaster, whining, complaining, and asking for more sweets. But with a low-sugar or no-sugar breakfast, like scrambled eggs and veggies and whole-grain toast, most kids will be calm, attentive, curious, and happy.

In addition to its effects on mood and energy levels, breakfast sets the tone for eating habits for the rest of the day. If kids hop onto the sugar roller coaster first thing in the morning, they will usually stay aboard all day long. One sugar high and crash fuels another. Kids can spend the whole day riding this cycle without realizing it. Breakfast with protein and fiber will solve the problem, providing steady energy throughout the day.

One problem: The older your kids get, the harder it can be to get them to eat *any* sort of breakfast. National data shows that more than 95 percent of kids ages two through five eat breakfast. However, this number falls to 90 percent for six-to-eleven-year-olds. In teens, those numbers go down again: only 76 percent of teen boys and 69 percent of teen girls eat breakfast. Whether it's an issue of time, personal preference, family finances, or a desire to diet, skipping breakfast hampers a child's academic performance and cognitive function, and can also nearly double the risk of becoming overweight. Skipping breakfast also leads to eating more carbohydrates and fat in the evenings. If you eat a balanced breakfast, you decrease the chances you'll binge on a huge, unhealthy meal for dinner. For kids of any age, the first important step is to incorporate breakfast into the daily routine.

The second step is to choose breakfast foods that keep blood glucose levels as steady as possible. Sweetened cereals, waffles or pancakes with syrup, muffins or other pastries, convenience items like Pop Tarts or breakfast bars, toast with jam, packets of sweetened instant oatmeal, apple or orange juice, and hot chocolate all create spikes in blood glucose levels. These spikes are followed by a crash, a state of low blood sugar that turns on your child's hunger and desire to eat again. When kids start their days with foods that are lower in sugar and higher in protein and fiber, they have better glycemic control, they experience increased fullness, and their brains are better able to regulate appetite and eating behavior.

I (Michael) once performed an experiment to test my own response to breakfast. I tried out three different breakfasts on three consecutive days: toast and marmalade, plain steel-cut oatmeal, and toast with two eggs (Figure 8). I wore a glucose monitor that measured my blood sugar over the course of the entire day. When I had toast and marmalade, I boarded the sugar roller coaster. My blood sugar rose quickly, peaked at about one hour after breakfast, dropped, and then after about two hours there was a second rise and fall. I went up and down that second "hill" because when glucose falls rapidly, there is a compensatory response. The body produces and releases more glucose into the circulation. When I had oatmeal for breakfast, the first spike wasn't as extreme, and the crash was not as severe, but it was still there and there

Figure 8: Michael's Blood Glucose Levels over 2.5 Hours after Three Different Breakfasts

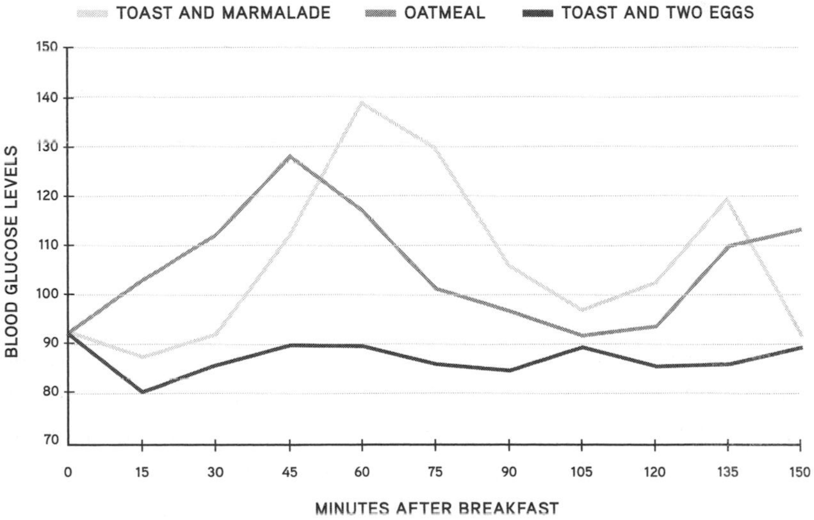

was still a second rise after about two hours. In contrast, the breakfast of toast with eggs gave me steady energy with no spike or crash. My blood glucose was stable and steady all morning. The difference was the protein and fat in the eggs that balanced out the carbohydrate in the toast and lowered the overall glycemic index of the breakfast.

We realize that breakfast can be the hardest meal of the day for parents. You're trying to manage everyone's taste preferences, get yourself and the kids dressed, and locate lost homework—all while keeping an eye on a clock that's quickly counting down the seconds. We're here for you with some easy ways your whole family can rethink breakfast.

The Cereal Fix

Kids love breakfast cereal, especially ones high in sugar. It's crunchy, sweet, and the boxes feature fun characters, secret codes for video games, and even small toys. It's a quick, easy solution that kids can often serve themselves. What's tricky about boxed cereal is not just the sugar content, but also the portion size that kids often eat. For example, even if the nutrition label on a box of cereal indicates that a serving is ¾ cup or 1 cup, kids will typically consume much more in a normal bowl of cereal, especially when they serve themselves. To test this at home, have your kids pour a bowl of cereal and measure the number of cups. You might discover that your kids are eating 2 cups, which is at least two servings. If the nutrition label indicates 10 grams of sugar per 1-cup serving, your child's bowl will contain 20 grams—or 5 teaspoons of added sugar, which is the total daily recommendation for a ten-year-old.

Eliminating sugary cereal is the best way to go, but if you just can't, then look for brands that have fewer than 3 grams of added sugar per serving. Try cutting the portion size by using smaller bowls and offering fruit toppings. In one study, ninety-one kids at a summer day camp were randomly sorted into two group. One group could choose from three high-sugar cereals; the other group chose from three low-sugar cereals. All the kids had free access to sliced bananas and strawberries and packets of sugar. Regardless of which group they were assigned to, children reported "liking" or "loving" their choice of cereal. But children in the high-sugar group ended up consuming almost *twice* as much cereal. Some of the children in the low-sugar group added sugar, but overall, they consumed about half as much sugar across the entire breakfast. Additionally, children in the low-sugar cereal group were much more likely to put fruit on their cereal. The bottom line? Kids will self-regulate, but that self-regulation will depend on what's put in front of them. Now there's news you can use! When serving cereal, keep it low in added sugar and have chopped fruit or berries available for toppings.

Adding protein to breakfast cereal is another useful strategy. This will help turn on the body's "feeling full" receptors. Protein reduces the impact of carbohydrates, which means kids will eat less and avoid an energy crash later. Cow's milk, whether whole or skim, has around 8 grams of protein per cup. If you are using a plant-based milk, choose carefully, as these products often have less protein and usually contain added sugars. Look for one with no added sugars and try adding chopped nuts or seeds on top of the cereal to increase the protein.

You can also serve cereal with yogurt instead of milk. Regular plain yogurt has around 8 grams of protein per cup, similar to milk. Unsweetened Greek yogurt is especially high in protein because it is strained: 1 cup has around 20 grams of protein. It can be a little tangy or sour for kids who are not used to it, but many kids enjoy it after an initial adjustment period, especially when they can top it with a cereal they like and some fresh fruit for natural sweetness and extra nutrients. This is also a great way to limit the portion of cereal, because the yogurt itself is very filling. Using yogurt instead of milk for cereal also provides beneficial probiotics. If your children can't eat dairy, try an unsweetened plant-based yogurt such as soy, coconut milk, or even almond milk yogurt, but check the label. Like the plant-based milks, they can have hidden sugars and a low protein value. If using a plant-based yogurt, add chopped nuts or seeds as a topping.

How Much Protein Does Your Child Need Each Day?

Daily protein requirements for children vary by age:

Age 2–3 years: 13g protein

Age 4–8 years: 19g protein

Age 9–13 years: 34g protein

Age 14–18 years: 52g protein (boys) or 46g protein (girls)

For reference, here are the protein contents of a few popular breakfast foods:

Greek yogurt, 1 cup: 20g

Plain yogurt, 1 cup: 8g

Cow's milk, 1 cup: 8g

Almonds, ¼ cup: 7g

Black beans, ½ cup: 7g

1 egg, large: 6g

Sausage, 1-oz. patty: 5g

The Oatmeal Fix

Oatmeal and other hot cereals have a healthy reputation, but be careful. Like cold cereals, most types of oatmeal are just big loads of carbohydrates that break down quickly to glucose. While oatmeal is more complex to break down than straight sugar, it can still usher kids onto the sugar roller coaster, especially if it is an instant variety or is topped with brown sugar, maple syrup, or other sweeteners. There are some ways to make your oatmeal truly healthful, however.

Skip the instant oats and go for steel-cut

The premade packets of instant oatmeal are often flavored and presweetened. Skip these. Even if they're not presweetened, the oats have been highly processed to make them ready to eat. Because they've been processed, they rate higher on the glycemic index, translating to a blast of energy and bigger spike in blood glucose levels. It's much better to cook the oats from scratch. The quick-cook (not instant) oats are okay in a pinch, but the Holy Grail of oatmeal is the steel-cut kind. Steel-cut oats are the cut-up oat grain (called a "groat"). They take longer to cook, but you can save time in the morning by soaking them overnight, which significantly reduces the cooking time. See our recipe on page 292 for a few different methods, including one that requires no cooking at all. You can also make steel-cut oats quickly in a pressure cooker or Instant Pot. Or simply make a batch at the start of the week and reheat single servings on subsequent days. We also like Scottish oats as a second-best option, which are stone-ground into smaller pieces so that they cook faster; even when cooked with water, they have a nice creamy texture and taste.

Add protein and sweeten with fruit

Just as with cold cereal, you'll need to balance the sugar and carbs in oatmeal with protein. Cooking oats in milk instead of water can help. And instead of the classic brown sugar or maple syrup as a sweetener, set out some fresh, frozen, or chopped dried fruits as toppings. They all have the advantage of adding fiber as well as vitamins and minerals to breakfast. Grace, who we introduced you to in Chapter 4, discovered a new favorite breakfast: oatmeal cooked with water and almond meal and topped with pecans and raspberries.

Make sure you check dried fruit for any added sugars, which are often used to sweeten tart fruits like cherries and cranberries. Keep in mind that all dried fruit contains concentrated sugar, even if it is naturally occurring. A rough target to follow is to use no more than ¼ cup per serving. Try distributing the naturally occurring sugars from dried fruits like raisins or chopped dates by cooking them with the oats. A simple apple or berry compote also makes a delicious topping for oatmeal (see Simple Fruit Compotes, page 339).

Try a savory porridge

Oatmeal or other hot cereals like grits or whole-grain rice cereal can easily be turned into a savory breakfast by adding a little butter or cheese, or by topping them with a fried egg. Traditional versions of savory rice porridge also include Chinese congee or Thai jok, which usually include chicken or ground pork and are topped with brightly flavored items like grated fresh ginger, cilantro, and green onion. We like to sprinkle hot cereals with furikake, which is a Japanese mixture of roasted seaweed, salt, and roasted sesame seeds that comes in a wide variety of flavors. Look for a brand that does not contain added sugars (e.g., Trader Joe's has one)—most do have a small amount (often ½ gram of sugar in ½ tablespoon), which is a whole lot less than if it was smothered with maple syrup. Introducing savory options can help broaden breakfast horizons and be useful in getting out of a sweet rut.

The Toast Fix

Toast is a quick breakfast option that can usually benefit from a healthy makeover. Start with a whole-grain bread with no added sugar. Sourdough breads can be a relatively good choice because they typically are made without added sugar. From this base, build your toppings wisely. Jam, jelly, or Nutella puts kids right on the sugar roller coaster. Even if the jam says "no added sugar," make sure to check the ingredient list for low-calorie sweeteners or fruit juice concentrates.

Instead, offer toppings that are full of protein, fiber, or healthy fat. Try ricotta cheese and grated lemon zest or a homemade fruit compote (see Simple Fruit Compotes on page 339). Other good options for toppings include avocado, unsweetened nut butters, hummus, smoked salmon, fried or scrambled eggs, cheese, or deli meat. Use the same strategy for bagels. Look for whole-grain bagels with no added sugar and top them with a source of protein like cream cheese or peanut butter. Bagels are bigger and denser than toast, with about the same amount of carbohydrates in three slices of bread, so consider mini-bagels or just half a bagel.

The Pancakes and Waffles Fix

Kids love pancakes or waffles for breakfast, but in addition to the sugar in the pancakes or waffles themselves, they tend to get drowned in maple syrup or covered with Nutella or chocolate chips. This sweet breakfast with no protein is a fun treat, but it can disrupt your child's energy levels throughout the day until bedtime. Try replacing the syrup with fruit, a fruit compote, or even non-sweetened whipped cream. One eight-year-old who did our 7-Day Challenge learned to sauté bananas in a little butter for a pancake topping. As the bananas caramelize in the pan, they release more of their natural sugars, making them a naturally sweet treat.

For protein, try toppings like unsweetened nut butter, ricotta cheese, or yogurt to go along with chopped fruit or berries. If you are making your own batter, you can increase the protein content by adding an extra egg, egg white, almond flour or another high-protein flour, or protein powder. Or you can serve a high-protein side dish like an egg or some sausage or lean Canadian bacon. Making crepes instead of pancakes or waffles also reduces the carbohydrate load: see our recipe for Three, Two, One . . . Crepes! (page 284). These work great with fruit toppings or savory toppings and make it easier to avoid maple syrup, as your family probably won't expect it as much as they do when you make pancakes or waffles.

What about those convenient toaster waffles that are so easy to grab-and-go? A serving of plain toaster waffles (2 waffles) has around 4 grams of added sugar (without the syrup), and less than 1 gram of fiber. They are not a smart choice. That's not to mention the added sugars from maple syrup that will likely get poured on top at 14 grams per tablespoon. Try replacing toaster waffles with whole-grain toast and adding some of the toppings suggested above to create a protein balance.

The Baked Goods Fix

Premade muffins, pastries, quick breads, and doughnuts are popular breakfast items, but they tend to be loaded with sugar. Your child might as well eat a slice of cake for breakfast. For example, a typical blueberry muffin from a coffee shop or bakery can easily contain 30 grams of sugar, little of which is coming from the blueberries. Cut large muffins in half to reduce the portion size and combine them with a protein like yogurt, milk, or an egg. Better yet, try making our Blueberry Banana Muffins (page 288), which contain no added sugars and a higher protein and fiber content than standard types.

The Breakfast Bar Fix

Most commercially produced breakfast bars, including granola and fruit bars, are marketed as healthy options with protein and vitamins. In reality, they contain high levels of added sugars. One package of Belvita Cranberry Orange Breakfast Biscuits, for example, contains 12 grams of sugar. Since they're not generally very filling and don't contain much protein, they may not satisfy a kid's appetite. You may find your kids wanting a second package, which doubles their sugar intake. One family we worked with had two children. Each of them ate up to three ZonePerfect Double Dark Chocolate Bars each morning. With 14 grams of sugar per bar, the kids were often eating more than their total daily sugar allowance at breakfast alone. Make your own using our recipe for granola thins (see Sugarproof Granola and Granola Thins, page 295), so you can control the sugar and add enough protein and fiber to make them balanced.

What about School Breakfasts?

Many kids eat breakfast at school, and the options can vary widely. You can help your children make smart choices by encouraging them to choose regular milk over chocolate or strawberry milk, whole fruit over juice, cereal with less sugar, and a protein such as egg or cheese.

Breakfast Options Based on Prep Time

NO TIME: GRAB-AND-GO OPTIONS

- Homemade Sugarproof muffins (prepared in advance; see Blueberry Banana Muffins, page 288)
- Sugarproof Granola and Granola Thins (prepared in advance, page 295)
- Overnight Steel-Cut Oats, Two Ways, cold version (prepared in advance in portable containers; page 292)

○ Fuss-Free Frittata (made in advance and eaten cold; page 279)

○ Other dinner leftovers that include protein and fiber

○ A hard-boiled egg (prepared in advance)

○ Whole or cut fruit (banana, apple, melon, berries) and a quick protein (e.g., a handful of nuts or a slice of cheese or a plain yogurt)

○ Rolled-up deli meat (no-added-sugar variety) with or without cheese

○ Whole-grain crackers with cheese or deli meat

5 MINUTES: QUICK BREAKFASTS

○ Breakfast cereal with fewer than 3 grams of sugar per serving with milk or yogurt and chopped fruit and/or berries

○ Toast topped with unsweetened nut or seed butter, avocado, cheese, ricotta, kefir/yogurt, fruit compote (see Simple Fruit Compotes, page 339), smoked salmon, deli meat, etc.

○ Plain yogurt topped with fruit, fruit compote (see Simple Fruit Compotes, page 339), and/or unsweetened cereal or Sugarproof Granola (see Sugarproof Granola and Granola Thins, page 295)

○ European-style breakfast with deli meats, cheeses, toast, vegetables like cucumber and tomatoes, ricotta, Swiss, or feta cheese

○ High protein smoothie made with whole fresh or frozen fruit and vegetables (optional), unsweetened milk of choice, and yogurt or a protein powder

10–15 MINUTES: QUICK-COOKING OR REHEATING

○ Fried, scrambled, or soft-boiled eggs and toast with the option of a sausage patty or Canadian bacon

○ Egg in a Basket (an egg cooked inside a piece of toast; page 281)

○ Popeye Scramble with Sweet Potato Toast (eggs scrambled with spinach; page 280)

○ Oatmeal cooked with milk of choice and topped with a protein like nuts or seeds or another savory topping

○ Dinner leftovers, reheated

○ Reheated crepes, pancakes, or waffles with choice of topping: fresh fruit, cheese, smoked salmon, etc.

○ Reheated frittata

○ Three, Two, One...Crepes! (page 284)

○ Fuss-Free Frittata (page 279)

○ Sugarproof muffins (see Blueberry Banana Muffins, page 288, and Apple Plum Muffins, page 290)

○ Traditional Japanese breakfast: Broiled fish of choice, miso soup, and rice

○ Any other cooked, international-style breakfasts of choice, such as pupusa or rice and beans

Expand Your Breakfast Horizons

If you've traveled outside the United States or have international friends, you've probably noticed that breakfast foods in other countries can be very different. Often, breakfast is just like any other meal, with protein and vegetables. In Japan, breakfast often includes miso soup and fish. In some European countries, breakfast features meats and cheeses as well as crunchy vegetables. Cucumbers, tomatoes, and feta cheese are popular in Greece and Turkey, while tamales are popular in Mexico. To expand your family's repertoire, ask your kids to help you research traditional breakfasts from around the world and find one of interest that is savory, not sweet. Once you research a breakfast, you can shop and prep for it, enjoy it together, and then talk about how it's different (*and* what your kids do and don't like about it).

Sugarproof Strategy #2: Ditch the Liquid Sugar

If your kids are drinking sweet drinks of any kind, including 100 percent fruit juice, then weaning them off this liquid sugar is the single most important dietary change you can make.

Fruit juice is often thought of as a breakfast staple, but it delivers a rapid and high dose of fructose. If you've worked to balance breakfast cereal or toast with protein to avoid a sugar crash, adding juice will spoil your efforts. Dr. Alaina Vidmar, a colleague at Children's Hospital Los Angeles, calls juice "an interesting drug." As she explains, after children are introduced to juice, they start consuming it in vast quantities and have a hard time giving it up. Parents often feel that juice is a healthier option than soda. But in fact, juice can be just as addictive and harmful.

Of course, there's no shortage of other sweet drinks for kids. Some are marketed for breakfast, some for sports, and some for all day long: Strawberry Quik. Chocolate milk. Frappuccinos. Sodas (regular or diet). Gatorade. Coconut water. If your kids are hooked on these drinks, you'll need some help. The goal is to help your child transition to water (plain or naturally flavored) as their primary beverage. A moderate amount of unsweetened milk, such as one or two glasses a day, is also usually fine for most children and even recommended, though it's best to consult with your pediatrician for specific guidance. Here are some tactics that will help you make the shift to reduce and maybe even eliminate liquid sugar.

Scratch soda and juice from your grocery list

The best way to cut back on sodas and sugary drinks is to stop buying them at the grocery store. Research shows that children and teens consume most of their soda or juice at home. If you don't bring them home, you have already cut back on consumption. Remember that we also do not recommend diet drinks that have artificial or other LCS in them.

Dilute, dilute, dilute

Instead of asking kids to give up sweet drinks cold turkey, you can wean kids from their sugar by gradually diluting them. The trick is using the right unsweetened mixer to dilute your children's favorite beverages. For soda, try plain sparkling water, club soda, or adding more ice. Many soda fountains feature unsweetened soda water as an option, which you can use to dilute the soda right at the fountain. Dilute juice or sports drinks with plain or sparkling water. Dilute flavored milk with plain. Add progressively more of the mixer until your children can give up the sweet drink and enjoy just the mixer (plain water, sparkling water, or milk) as a beverage. For coffee drinks or tea, the trick is to gradually cut back on the sugar or sweetener until kids develop a new taste for the less sweet drink. For drinks that are made from sugared or sugar-free powdered mix, like Nesquik, Kool-Aid, or Crystal Light, use less powder until you arrive at plain water or milk.

Keep water handy and make it appealing

Make plain water the default drink at home, with meals, and at school. If your refrigerator does not dispense cold water, keep large glass bottles or pitchers of water in the refrigerator. Keeping cold water in the fridge means it's always ready for mealtimes. If your tap water doesn't taste very good, consider investing in a basic water filter pitcher like a Brita or an in-home water filter or reverse osmosis system. The investment you make in the water your family can drink at home will pay for itself as you wean your kids off sugary drinks, both in their improved health and your reduced grocery bill.

Before leaving for an outing, prepare water bottles to take with you so that there will be less temptation to buy other drinks while you're out. Let your kids choose a fun, colored, stainless steel, insulated water bottle for school. For younger kids, make sure to keep portable cups or child-friendly water bottles accessible to them no matter where they are playing. These bottles will keep water tasting cool and fresh and will also be good for the environment by reducing single-use plastic water bottles.

Add flavor without sugar

Kids who are used to sweetened drinks often crave flavor when switching to drinking plain water. Try making pitchers of naturally flavored water to keep in your refrigerator. You can easily add sliced citrus like lemon, lime, orange, or grapefruit or other fruit like apples, kiwi, berries, watermelon, or even sliced cucumber or fresh mint. You can also try adding individual pieces of frozen fruit to water bottles for school or sports practice. If your kids like sparkling water, look for a brand that's flavored but unsweetened. Make sure you check the label to avoid both sugar and LCS. You can also look into a machine like a SodaStream that carbonates plain water with a charged cartridge of CO_2. Your kids will have fun making their own sparkling water fruit drinks with fresh or frozen fruit.

Take time for tea

Warm or iced tea is a great way to enjoy a beverage socially with family or friends instead of ordering a sweet, coffee-based drink. Herbal teas, also called *tisanes*, are "teas" that contain no tea leaves or caffeine but include flowers, botanicals, and even spices and bits of citrus peel. There are many types of flavorful herbal teas, and you can involve everyone in picking out new types to try that taste good with no added sugar or sweetener. They are usually good both iced and hot. Teas are also a great option for kids who want to go to the coffee shop with their friends. Most coffee shops carry a wide variety of tea, which means that your teen can enjoy time with their friends and skip the sugar without feeling left out. Just be sure to avoid teas with caffeine, especially before bedtime.

Drink wisely when eating out

Sometimes it can be hard to resist sweet options at cafés or restaurants, especially if it is a special occasion. Try ordering one drink to share and pour it into a few glasses, then add water. My (Emily's) kids like to order plain sparkling water at restaurants, and even though it is an extra expense, it helps them feel that they've ordered something special. When at a café and ordering a flavored coffee drink, ask for fewer pumps of syrup or sweetener or fewer scoops of powder. Try the drink at 75 percent sweetness, then work your way down to see if 25 percent sweetness is acceptable.

Watch out for premade smoothies

Premade smoothies or juices can seem like a simple way to add nutrients to your children's diet. But even green smoothies or vegetable-based smoothies can be very high in added sugar or hidden sweeteners. Even if they're labeled "all plant based" and "natural—with no added sugar," check the ingredient list. More often than not, you'll find ingredients like juice, fruit juice concentrate, agave, or monk fruit used as sweeteners. Yes, your kids may be getting a few leaves of spinach or kale in that green smoothie, but they may also be getting the equivalent of the juice of three apples without the fiber. If your kids love smoothies, try making them at home with fresh or frozen fruit, leafy greens or other vegetables, and yogurt or protein powder, using either water or an unsweetened milk of choice as the liquid. See our recipes for smoothies on pages 298 and 335.

Sugarproof Strategy #3: Avoid Fructose

If your family gives up sweetened drinks, they're avoiding the biggest typical source of fructose. But there are other ways that unhealthy amounts of fructose can creep into children's diets. To maintain a lower-fructose diet in your house, avoid any products sweetened with high-fructose corn syrup, fruit juice concentrates, agave syrup, or fructose itself. Each of these sugars has a high fructose component. As you scan ingredient lists, also be wary of anything that says "fruit juice sweetened" or "fruit sugar."

As we discussed in Chapter 3, some kinds of sugar have an undeserved reputation for being healthier or more natural. Ultimately, they're all still sugar—at least, in terms of how your body and brain react to them. And sugar that is made up of a higher percentage of fructose than glucose can have more damaging effects. The table "Sugar According to Fructose Content" will help you spot the sugar products that are highest in fructose.

Sugar According to Fructose Content

SUGAR*	FRUCTOSE	GLUCOSE	COMMENTS
Fructose; crystalline fructose	100%	0%	Often labeled as "fruit sugar" and as a "healthy sugar." Avoid any product listing fructose as an ingredient.
High-fructose corn syrup	55–90%	10–42%	Avoid.
Agave syrup	90%	10%	Sugar profile varies but typically very high in fructose. Avoid.
Apple or pear juice concentrate	70%	30%	Actual composition varies but typically high in fructose. Avoid.
Honey	50.5%	44.5%	Adds flavor, some trace nutrients, and has medicinal properties; fructose and glucose ratios can vary. Use sparingly.
Date sugar/date syrup	50%	50%	Sugar profile can vary quite a bit depending on type of date, with some higher in glucose and others higher in fructose, adds flavor, can contain fiber depending on manufacturing. Use sparingly.
Coconut sugar	50%	50%	Sugar profile can vary quite a bit; adds flavor; contains small amounts of fiber; sustainable to grow. Use sparingly.
Sucrose/sugar/ brown sugar	50%	50%	Also known as table sugar and includes products like raw sugar or cane sugar. Use sparingly.
Maple syrup	48.5%	51.5%	Adds flavor and trace nutrients; amounts of fructose and glucose can vary. Use sparingly.
Grape juice concentrate	40%	60%	The actual sugar profile varies, so we suggest avoiding grape juice concentrate whenever possible.

Note: We simplified the table by dividing any sucrose in these sugars into half glucose and half fructose. Also note the values in this table are estimates, as the actual percentages can vary based on the exact sources.

Whole fruits contain fructose, but, as we've mentioned, they generally do not cause problems, provided your children don't eat enormous quantities all at once. That's because the health effects of fructose are related to how quickly it is ingested; how fast it enters the bloodstream; and whether other nutrients and components, like fiber, are present in the fruit.

To better evaluate just how *bad* the fructose is in fruit and fruit products—that is, how fast it will enter the bloodstream—we've created the Fructose Index. The faster the fructose is broken down and absorbed into the bloodstream, the more likely it will have detrimental effects on the body in both the short and long term.

Take a look at four preparations of apples to see how fructose is liberated. A good rule of thumb is "Eat fruit, don't drink it."

The Fructose Index

LOW FRUCTOSE INDEX/ LOW RISK	**Whole apple**	Optimal because you get all the benefits of the fiber and nutrients in the apple and the fructose is slowly released during digestion, limiting its potential damaging effects on the liver. Also, typical serving sizes (such as a whole apple) contain a lot less sugar than in a typical serving size of apple juice.
	Blended apple (as in a smoothie or applesauce)	When blending or pureeing fruit, the fiber is still retained, which helps slow the absorption of the fructose. Note that many commercial brands of applesauce do not include the peel. Look for an applesauce that is made with the peel or make your own.
	100% apple juice, including fresh squeezed	Juicing apples frees the fructose from the fibrous cells and eliminates the fiber in the process. Some of the healthy micronutrients of the apple might be retained, but juicing essentially creates highly concentrated fructose that makes it more rapidly available for processing by the liver, where it can be converted to fat.
HIGH FRUCTOSE INDEX/HIGH RISK	**Apple juice drink made with high-fructose corn syrup**	Fructose is free in solution and easily available for rapid uptake from the gut and absorption into the blood for immediate delivery to the liver for conversion to fat.

Beyond choosing whole fruits over juice, some fruits are lower in fructose than others, including berries, citrus, banana, and kiwi. It's okay for kids to eat the fruits that are higher in fructose, such as apples, pears, mango, watermelon, and grapes, as long as they aren't having excessive amounts all at once. We definitely don't recommend eating three apples or an entire bunch of grapes in one sitting. Generally we recommend no more than two to three servings of fruit per day, but not all at once.

Sugarproof Strategy #4: Use Snacks to Your Advantage

You pick your children up from school and they don't even greet you. Instead, they say, "What's for snack?" Even if you have something nutritious to give them, they scarf it down and declare they are still hungry. One snack turns into two, and then three. It's easy for the snack situation to get out of hand. Know that you are not alone here.

- 96 percent of children consume at least 1 snack per day;

- 50 percent of children consume 2 or 3 snacks per day;

- The popularity of snacking is on the rise, especially in younger kids. Children ages two to six are the highest snack consumers (2.75 per day), an amount that doubled between 1977 and 2006;

- In younger kids, snacks constitute 30 percent of daily energy, which is enough to make up a breakfast, lunch, or dinner!

Kids, especially younger children, get hungry and need a snack between meals. The issue isn't just about the quality of the snack but also the amount of the snack and the timing. If snacks are more like balanced mini-meals or contain fresh fruits and vegetables, they're a fine option to fill up growing bodies and keep moods and energy even. Chips, cookies, crackers, granola bars, and processed fruit snacks are all choices that take up room in a child's diet that could otherwise be filled with healthier options. Ultimately, snack time can either be a prime chance to add nutrients to your children's diets or a major missed window of opportunity. Here are some tactics for making snacks work for you, not against you:

Seize the moment

There are times in the day when your children are genuinely hungry, such as after school or after sports practice. You know that they haven't eaten for a few hours and have expended energy. Here's a chance for you to offer something healthy. Don't waste the moment with cookies or a commercially processed granola bar that is full of sugar.

Recognize boredom and other triggers

There are other times when your child is not actually hungry but wants to snack out of boredom. When food is out on the kitchen counter or in other easy-to-reach places, it's tempting for everyone. Snacking becomes merely something mindless to do while watching TV or playing on the computer. If your child asks for a snack, or your teen is looking in the refrigerator or freezer for something to eat, propose an alternative activity like going outside, practicing music lessons, doing homework, or contacting a friend. Or offer a simple drink like water or herbal tea—your kids may be thirsty instead of hungry.

Prepare healthy snacks at home

Research shows that most snacking occurs at home, which is good news: It gives parents more influence over what their children are eating. Stock your pantry with Sugarproof snacks or prep them in advance. When you have healthy snacks on hand, they're also easy to drop into a backpack or lunch bag.

Involve the kids in prep

Kids love to get involved in kitchen tasks like washing vegetables or threading cherry tomatoes, basil, and mozzarella onto toothpicks for little Caprese skewers. When you have more time, spend some with your kids researching, choosing, and making snacks in advance like our Crispy Chickpea Snacks (page 316), Tamari-Roasted Sunflower Seeds (page 318), Easy No-Bake Energy Bites (page 319), or granola thins (see Sugarproof Granola and Granola Thins, page 295).

Serve a starter before the meal

Think of a pre-dinner snack as a "starter" for the main meal. If your kids are asking for snacks while you are cooking, consider prepping the vegetable component of the meal first and giving it to them as an appetizer. Or simply let them snack on raw vegetables like carrot sticks, cucumber slices, or cherry tomatoes to take the edge off their hunger.

Be flexible about mealtimes

Are your children asking for a snack at 11:00 a.m.? Is it possible instead to serve lunch? If after-school snack time is getting out of hand, can you move dinnertime earlier? This can be difficult with work schedules, but for some families, it is possible to shift mealtimes. In other cases, it may be worth it to give your kids dinner earlier than the rest of the family eats, especially for younger kids. While research definitely supports the notion that having the family eat together promotes more balanced meals, you need to evaluate your own situation. If kids can eat dinner soon after they return home from school, a parent can still sit with them regardless of whether or not the parent eats. Shifting the timing can reduce their demands for snacks, help them eat a better dinner, and also allow for an earlier bedtime if you're also trying to make a sleep adjustment.

More quantity at meals

If your kids are asking for snack after snack, it could be that they aren't eating enough at mealtime. For example, if you are packing only half of a sandwich at lunch, consider a full-size sandwich. Teenagers may even want or need two sandwiches or extra side items in their lunches, especially if they are athletes or stay at school for extended hours.

Reconsider snacks during screen time

Whether it's their favorite show or scheduled video gaming time, snacking during screen time can easily turn into mindless eating. If you are going to let your kids snack while watching a program or gaming, give them something that you don't mind they eat a lot of, such as cucumbers or carrot slices. We all know how fast a bag of cookies can disappear . . . and surprisingly, veggies will often magically disappear just as quickly.

Sugarproof Strategy # 5: Choose Sweet Treats Wisely

We are all for the occasional dessert or treat, but the trick is knowing how to enjoy it and to be careful about *when* and *how much*. As a parent, you can wisely time when kids have sweets and keep them to a reasonable portion. Eating sweets on an empty stomach is going to pack a bigger sugar punch than dessert after a meal when the stomach is already full and digestion will be slower.

One way to shift the thinking, especially for kids, is to think of sweets as dessert—not a snack. When you have already eaten a well-balanced meal, enjoying a small dessert shouldn't cause a major spike in blood sugar. If you have that same treat on an empty stomach, you would likely notice its effect. If you encourage sweets only after a meal, kids are less hungry and will eat less, ideally just a few bites. They'll also be more open to a much smaller portion or even sharing. It is important to have a short gap between the meal and the dessert to allow appetite signals and feelings of fullness to kick in. So a good time for a sweet treat would be fifteen to twenty minutes after a meal.

Portions sizes are very important when it comes to dessert. Children who serve themselves can end up taking a bigger portion if there is a bigger amount available. As a parent, you set the tone for the portion size of dessert, and portion sizes influence eating behavior. Research shows that children who are offered a larger portion size will consume more food compared to when they are offered a standard portion size. One way to avoid this situation is to offer "mini-desserts" when you are going to have them at home. In Michael's house, we sometimes have what we call mini-D: cookies, cake, ice cream, or other treats served in small portions on small plates, and often accompanied with herbal tea. This strategy has become second nature in the Goran house. Everyone is happy with a smaller portion and, most important, it reduces the *expectation* that dessert will be served in large portions. Smaller desserts also create a great opportunity to teach kids about mindful eating. Encourage them to slow down and enjoy each bite, thinking about the flavors and textures to increase their enjoyment.

Sometimes it can be especially hard to control portion sizes, such as when you are at a social gathering. If there is a dessert buffet where kids can take as much as they want of a larger dish, try to establish a norm for portion sizes. As children get older, they are more susceptible to food cues in the environment and less responsive to internal hunger cues. By establishing a habit of small portion sizes for desserts, you will help your children keep sugar in moderation and allow them to more accurately assess hunger no matter what type of situation they are in.

Need some more tips for keeping portion sizes under control?

• Share desserts when eating out.

• If baking cookies or other treats at home, freeze some to have another week instead of having them two nights in a row, or share some with friends or neighbors.

• Instead of a whole batch of a favorite recipe, make half.

- Portion desserts onto individual plates or dishes in the kitchen rather than bringing a whole cake or other large item to the table.

- Use smaller plates or serving dishes so that portions don't look overly small. Research shows that serving food on small plates can improve portion control in children (and adults).

- Request a smaller portion if eating out or at a friend's house.

Sugarproof Strategy #6:
Set Guidelines for the Major Culprits

You have already instilled some basic rules in your children, such as "play nicely with others" and "always try your hardest." You may have some other rules in your home, too, like "no taking food to your room" or "no drinks next to the computer," or "if it's dirty, put it in the dishwasher." Have you considered some basic rules you might teach around sugar? In his book *Food Rules: An Eater's Manual*, the journalist Michael Pollan presents simple and memorable rules such as "Eat Food. Not Too Much. Mostly Plants," which have helped many people re-evaluate their food choices and instill an internal voice that helps guide them in making food decisions.

No matter whether your parenting style is easygoing or strict, you can give your kids a variety of clear rules for sugar consumption. If you focus on positive, supportive rules and not negative policing, you'll find that soon these new guidelines will become second nature. You do not have to follow them every single minute of your family's time together, but they can provide a helpful framework for decisions.

Studies show that kids who are raised in houses with healthy food rules make healthier food choices away from home. For example, researchers from Stanford collected data from 1,246 high schoolers in San Francisco and asked them to choose two snacks from an offering of ten different options that ranged in nutritional quality. The results showed that those who reported having at least one healthy eating rule at home (such as allowing junk food only on special occasions or expecting that a vegetable will be eaten with dinner) were almost two times more likely to choose a healthier snack.

Families who have tried our 7-Day and 28-Day Challenges have found that adopting sugar-related guidelines is very effective in changing old habits and establishing new norms around sugar. The guidelines might be different for each family depending on specific circumstances; it was their very existence that made them effective. Maybe you'll have dessert only on weekends. Or maybe you will decide not to buy ice cream to keep at home, but instead go out once a month for ice cream as a family. You can guide children with rules, depending on their problem areas. If your nine-year-old consumes candy at every opportunity, maybe it's time to set a guideline like no candy during the week, or no candy after 4:00 p.m. With a rule like this, your kids might look forward to the weekend, maybe talking about it midweek. But after a few weeks, they will likely have forgotten about the candy and won't even bring it up. Setting guidelines can be a smart way to break the vicious cycle of sugar and its activation of the internal reward system.

The rule that families we work with find the most helpful is "one treat per day." This guideline doesn't mean you *must* have one treat per day—it means that if there has already been one treat today, then you won't have any other treats. This strategy works well for younger children because it allows them to control their own decisions. I (Emily) raised both of my boys with this rule. By the time they each reached age three, they had internalized it and are now comfortable with it. For example, they know that if we go to a morning event and they choose to have a treat that's offered there, then that's it for the day. Anything else can be enjoyed on another day. It's a great way to stick to just one a day for a child whose entire world is inundated with ads and opportunities to want sugar. Once most children know the guidelines, they're less likely to put up a big fuss about it, especially when they know those guidelines are enforced.

Here are some other Sugarproof guidelines you could incorporate, based on whatever seems to be a major issue in your house:

- No drinking soda or other sweet drinks in the house

- Dessert at weekend nights only or one mini dessert during the week and one on the weekend or on a special occassion

- Sweets only after a meal

- No buying prepackaged cookies, but instead baking cookies as a family once a month

- Savory after-school snacks instead of sweet ones

- Whole fruit at breakfast instead of juice

- If ordering a coffee/tea drink, ask for fewer pumps of sugar/syrup

Sugarproof Strategy #7: Work a Restaurant Menu like a Pro

How often do you open a restaurant menu and realize there aren't many healthy choices? But with a few tricks up your sleeve, you—and your kids—can become pros at creative ordering, whether at a restaurant, a take-out spot, or the local coffee shop. You'll be able to teach kids that there are usually more options available to them than just nuggets, fries, and a sugar bomb of a drink.

Know where the sugar hides

Certain dishes are more likely to have added sugar than others. Take a typical teriyaki chicken bowl or a sushi dinner with rolls drizzled with eel sauce or ponzu sauce. These healthy-sounding choices could easily contain up to 40 grams of sugar per serving, thanks to the sauces and/or the sugar that's added to the sushi rice. The table below can give you some guidelines for items where sugar may lurk when you order out.

CUISINE	RED LIGHT: Things That Tend to Have Added Sugar	YELLOW LIGHT: Choices That May or May Not Have Added Sugar or Smaller Amounts of Sugar	GREEN LIGHT: Choices that Tend to Be Free of Added Sugars
Mexican	Horchata, aguas frescas, mole sauce	Salsa, flour tortillas	Corn tortillas, guacamole, grilled meats like fajitas or carne asada, beans
Chinese	Dishes with sauces like sweet and sour, black bean, oyster, or orange glaze	Meat and vegetable stir-fries with garlic or ginger	Steamed brown rice, fried rice, steamed vegetables
American	Hamburger buns, ketchup, breaded proteins like chicken nuggets or fish sticks, salad dressings like French or honey mustard, barbecue sauce, coleslaw, baked beans	Marinated meats	Hamburger without the bun, grilled meats or fish, salads with oil and vinegar dressing
Thai	Pad Thai, pad kee mao, satay sauce or other dipping sauces	Curry dishes, stir fry dishes with sauces, soups, spring rolls	Steamed brown rice, steamed vegetables
Japanese	Sushi; sweet sauces like teriyaki, ponzu, or eel sauce	Noodle soups	Miso soup, sashimi or grilled fish, steamed brown rice, edamame
Italian		Tomato sauce for pizza or pasta (especially at chain restaurants), pizza dough (especially at chains), breadsticks	Risotto, pasta with vegetables or seafood, salads, second courses like grilled meats or fish
Vietnamese	Marinated meats, noodle dishes with dressing/sauce, dipping sauces	Curry dishes, stir-fries with sauces, spring rolls, pho soup	Steamed brown rice, steamed vegetables

Be wary of the kids' menu

Meals marketed specifically to kids are often full of fat, salt, and sugar. Too often a sweet drink and a dessert are built into the menu, making it harder to say no. But if you learn to order wisely, you can still save money and control the sugar intake. If you are going to order from the kids' menu, consider asking for water or milk instead of juice, lemonade, or soda, or dilute them down to share. Or you can give your child the choice of the sweet drink or the dessert, but not both. You can also simply ask the waiter to skip bringing the dessert. And as a last option, you can split a sugary kid's meal between two kids and add a healthier side dish to supplement it.

Check out the side dishes and starters

Sometimes appetizers and side dishes are just the right size for kids and can work as their meal. Try appetizers like chicken satay (minus any sweet dipping sauces) or other grilled meats on a stick, hummus with pita, or a soup. Side dishes can be great, too, such as a salad, steamed or sautéed vegetables, a baked sweet potato, or beans.

Order family style

Sharing dishes among family members can open up options for eating well. If you have two kids, you can order one main dish for them to share instead of getting each of them a kid's meal, skipping the sweet drink and dessert that likely come with the kid's meal. You can fill in gaps by ordering extra vegetable side dishes or salads if needed, and everyone can share these as well. If it is an occasion that calls for a special dessert, order just one (or two for a larger family) for everyone to share.

Don't be shy about asking

Do you see something on the menu that you are interested in, but you know that it probably has a lot of sugar? Maybe it's grilled meat with barbecue sauce or salad with a honey-mustard dressing. Don't be afraid to ask for more information and an eventual substitution. Ask for sauce on the side, no sauce at all, or a different sauce altogether. Sometimes

I (Emily) order Indian takeaway with my family. We ask for no added sugar in the curry, and the restaurant is happy to oblige.

Beat the buffet

Buffets pose special challenges. Since you're already paying a set price, you often feel you need to get the most for your money. Most kids want to try everything—especially the desserts—which can make it harder for you to limit their choices. However, there are some ways you can help your young child choose wisely, even in the face of a real sugar smorgasbord. To help navigate this situation, treat the buffet as consisting of multiple courses. Explain that all of the sweet items fall under the dessert course. This tactic is especially useful for breakfast buffets where kids are immediately drawn to sweet items like pastries or waffles with syrup. You can help avoid overdoing it with these if you explain to kids that these fall into the "dessert" category. First identify a protein to eat, such as scrambled eggs. From there, see if there are other healthy items to add in, like some fruit or a complex carbohydrate like plain oatmeal, unsweetened cereal, or whole-grain toast. Finally, after your child has had a decent meal, they can pick one of the sweet items to try or sample a smaller portion of two items, sharing with other family members.

Start Early: Sugarproof during Pregnancy and Early Infant Feeding

Maybe some of these strategies don't apply to you at the moment. Maybe you are expecting your first child or have a baby who doesn't eat solids yet. But it's never too early to start Sugarproofing your children. Protect them from the effects of sugars early on, starting during pregnancy, during early feeding, and during weaning to solids.

Pregnancy

Because weight gain is a natural part of pregnancy, it's a common misconception that it doesn't matter if what you eat is particularly healthy or not. It does matter, both for you and for the baby. But pregnancy is tough, and cravings and nausea can get in the way of making healthy food choices. Think about filling up the extra calories you need for your baby's growth with foods that are nutritious—and are free of added sugars and other sweeteners. Kate, a mom from San Francisco, was five months pregnant with her second daughter when she participated in our 7-Day Challenge. She had been craving dairy and had fallen into the habit of making herself a milkshake with vanilla ice cream each night. Thanks to the challenge, she changed this routine and started having a big cup of frothed milk with vanilla extract or fruit.

Breastfeeding

Breastfeeding is the most effective way to share immune benefits, nutrition, and numerous other benefits with your newborn child. Science is finding new evidence every day that it contributes to brain development and protects from a variety of health problems, including future childhood obesity and liver damage. However, breastfeeding can also be a challenge for some women when it doesn't seem to happen as naturally as it should.

If you are able to breastfeed, we recommend staying with it for at least six months with a target of one year or more. In one of our previous studies, kids who were breastfed for at least twelve months had lower levels of obesity than those breastfed for less than twelve months. And this extended breastfeeding protected kids even if they were later drinking a lot of sugary beverages. If you are able to breastfeed, it is important to consider that what you eat and drink influences the quality of your milk. Fructose can be passed from mother to baby via breast milk, so it is important to limit the amount of added sugar, and especially fructose, in your own diet while you are breastfeeding. Watch out for supplemental foods marketed to breastfeeding moms, like lactation cookies, which are typically high in sugar; in addition, there is no real evidence that they improve milk production.

Formula Feeding

Not all new mothers are able to breastfeed, and some choose not to. Others supplement feedings with formula for a wide variety of reasons. Most infant formulas have some form of sugar in them;

it is necessary for the baby's growth. It's the type of sugar that matters. Formulas that most closely match human breast milk contain lactose, which is the best option for babies. If your baby is not able to digest lactose (in infant formula, it comes from cow's milk), talk with your pediatrician. He or she should be able to help you find the best formula profile in terms of sugar. Be aware that some lactose-free formulas are sweetened with corn syrup solids, which are broken down to pure glucose, or, worse, with cane sugar, which the body breaks down into fructose and glucose. Avoid these whenever possible. Babies are not fully equipped to handle fructose, and the fructose itself may cause digestive problems if it is not absorbed. If any of it is absorbed, the fructose can wreak havoc with your infant's metabolism, causing problems such as fatty buildup in the liver, accelerated synthesis of new fat cells, and disruption of healthy appetite regulation. Also, some of these formulas are lactose reduced, which means they could be lacking in galactose, which is a vital sugar for infant brain development.

Weaning

Products marketed to parents for weaning their babies are usually full of added sugars, in particular fruit juice concentrates. These may sound healthy, as they are "fruit juice sweetened" and "all natural," but they contain fructose and other added sugars that simply have no place in a baby's diet. Juices program your child's body to want more sugar. Additionally, their sugar load can begin a cycle of organ damage as the liver works overtime to process the fructose that's delivered directly to the bloodstream. If you give sugar at this stage of development, you are buying your children a ticket for the sugar roller coaster they can ride all through childhood.

When transitioning your baby to solids, try to stay away from any products with added sugars in them, including teething biscuits, baby foods, and snacks. We suggest skipping any products that contain fruit juice concentrates, like pouches or jars of fruit and vegetable purees, flavored yogurts, or sweetened rice cakes. Remember that fruit juice concentrates are forms of added sugar, and particularly harmful ones at that, given their high fructose content. Also resist the urge to give your baby juice of any type, even if it is 100 percent juice and even if it is watered down.

With these seven Sugarproof strategies, it will be easier for your family to reduce added sugars. It will be easier to maintain the changes for the long term, too. You might find that these strategies alone give your family the boost it needs to reduce sugar. But if you'd like a jump start, or if you like having a plan to follow, read on. We'll show you how to put our 7-Day and 28-Day Challenges into place. The 7-Day Challenge asks your family to give up all added sugar, but just for one week, and the 28-Day Challenge allows families to reduce sugar gradually and to choose their priorities for sugar reduction. As you read and learn more, you can choose the one that most appeals to you, or you can try both. Either way, you're on the road to new, healthier habits for your children.

> To view the scientific references cited in this chapter, please visit us online at sugarproofkids.com/bibliography.

CHAPTER EIGHT

The 7-Day No-Added-Sugar Challenge: Sugarproof in One Week

If you want to reboot your family's diet quickly, try the 7-Day Challenge. In this plan, your family will give up all added sugar for a week. It's a big change for most families, but it works. This is not meant to be a diet per se that we expect you to stick to for the long term. Instead, think of this as an exercise you can do as a family to raise awareness about the extent of sugar in your household, identify sources of everyday foods with hidden sugars and find alternative replacements, and see how it feels to eliminate added sugars from the diet. Families who have completed this challenge have learned to appreciate the extent of hidden sugars in everyday foods and have been surprised at how quickly their children adjust to life without sugar. This short period of elimination will refresh palates and provide new appreciation for the flavor of food and drinks that haven't been sweetened. Families also report that cutting out sugar can dramatically stabilize up-and-down moods in a very short period of time. The 7-Day Challenge is designed to break old habits around sugar and yield positive results in just one week.

In this one-week program, we'll give you strategies for success and also prepare you for a few of the things you may experience, such as the symptoms of sugar withdrawal or resistance from your kids. The very best thing about the one-week plan is that it's here for you whenever you need it and can be repeated at any time. It's a good way to begin the Sugarproof process, teach your kids new habits, or reset your family's sugar intake whenever you feel you have been overdoing it. It's also a perfect way to recover from the sugar overload of holidays like Halloween or Christmas.

Is This Challenge Right for Your Family?

To help you decide if this 7-Day Challenge is right for you and your family, ask yourself these questions:

- Have you recently received alarming news from your pediatrician about your child's health?
- Do you want to determine whether there's a connection between your children's sugar intake and their health and mood problems?
- Have you recently been overdoing it with sugar, perhaps in the wake of a holiday?
- Are you looking to reset the entire family's health before school starts or in time for summer vacation?
- Are you and your family motivated by a good challenge?
- Do your kids respond better to change when it happens completely and quickly?
- Do you want to see immediate results before you commit to the long term?

If you answered "yes" to any of these questions, this short-term challenge could be right for you. If your family is more likely to respond to small changes that you phase in over time, and if there are no major health problems that you want to address right away, the 28-Day Challenge was made for you. You can find it starting on page 229.

Can One Week Really Make a Difference?

The short answer is *absolutely*. Surprisingly, even one week of no sugar can have a positive impact on health and metabolism. Parents report that their kids act less stressed, angry, anxious, and sad. If they're under a pediatrician's care, they may see improvement in their glucose levels or other blood tests. In a series of studies at the University of San Francisco, children were put on low-sugar diets for nine days. Even over this short period of time, the kids showed significant improvements in metabolic health related to type 2 diabetes, fatty liver disease, and cardiovascular disease.

We can't promise that the 7-Day Challenge will always be easy. Giving up sugar and sweeteners can be uncomfortable, especially in the first few days. But what we do know is that when families stick with the challenge, they feel better. As the diets and meals change, kids and adults feel fuller for longer because their blood sugar levels are more stable. Kids beg for fewer snacks and won't have as many "hangry" episodes or meltdowns. Kids will eat better at mealtimes, and bedtimes should be easier.

The 7-Day Challenge Step by Step

The 7-day plan is broken into nine steps, which we will walk you through.

- Know the "Rules"
- Get the Gang on Board
- Get Everyone Motivated
- Pick Your Week
- Check Everyday Staples for Hidden Sugars
- Create Your Personalized 7-Day Menu
- Shop and Prep Wisely

- Monitor and Troubleshoot
- Evaluate Next Steps

Taken step by step, the challenge becomes much easier.

Step 1: Know the "Rules"

In the 7-Day Challenge, your family won't eat any added sugar. Because added sugar is everywhere, it helps to identify the foods that are out during this week, as well as the foods that are in.

WHAT'S OUT:

- Any sugars or sweeteners that you use at home to add to foods during preparation are out for this week. This includes table sugar that you might have in a sugar bowl, honey in a jar, or brown sugar you keep around for your morning oatmeal.

- Natural-sounding sweeteners like fruit juice concentrate, honey, agave syrup, coconut sugar, and maple syrup are still sugar. They're out.

- Any packaged foods with any added sugar are also out. Yogurt, salad dressing, barbecue sauce, pasta sauce, cereals or bars, and many other prepared foods often contain added sugar and are out.

- Low-calorie sweeteners are out, whether it's Splenda in your morning coffee or diet sodas. Keep an eye out for "natural sweeteners" like stevia or monk fruit, which are also out for this week.

- Check product labels closely; even if a product says "no artificial sweeteners" or "no added sugar," it might still contain LCS.

- No fruit juice, even if it's 100 percent juice from the grocery or fresh squeezed at home. Coconut water is also out. Smoothies made at home using whole fruits are allowed. Watch out for commercially made smoothies, which usually contain juice, fruit juice concentrates, or other added sugars.

- Any other beverages with sugar or sweeteners are out. This means sports drinks, energy drinks, coffee drinks, iced tea, or sodas—both regular and diet.

What about Your Glass of Wine?

Can parents who are participating in the challenge have alcoholic beverages in moderation? We don't think it is a problem to have a drink or two during the challenge week, but keep in mind that alcohol adds empty calories to your diet and can also contribute sugar. Ciders are similar to juice and can contain significant amounts of sugar, so we recommend avoiding them. Some of the sweeter-tasting wine varieties can contain added sugar, and this is hard to ascertain from the label. For this reason, try to select dry varieties. For cocktails, avoid using juices, sugary sodas, or tonic as mixers. (Club soda is fine.) Also many premade mixes, premade cocktails, and bottled or canned specialty drinks are full of added sugar, so avoid them if possible.

WHAT'S IN:

- The only sweeteners allowed in this challenge are whole fruits. You can sweeten a smoothie with a banana or a date, or top a bowl of oatmeal with fresh or unsweetened dried fruit.

- Eating whole fruits is fine, but don't let your kids eat too much all at once. Around two to three servings a day of fruit is recommended. A serving of fresh fruit is one whole piece of a small fruit like an apple or a banana, 1 cup of cut fruit like melon or mango, or ½ cup of unsweetened dried fruit.

- Don't overdo it on dried fruit. Even when dried fruit doesn't contain added sugar, its natural sugars become very concentrated. And since dried fruit is not as filling, it's easy to overeat. An entire apricot is much more filling because of the water content than a handful of dried apricots, which might be the equivalent of five apricots or more.

- The natural sugars in milk and dairy products are fine as long as you check the list of ingredients for any other possible added sugars. New food labels being introduced in 2020–2021 are required to list any added sugars separately, which will make this task easier (see Chapter 2 for more information), but if a food label does not clearly distinguish added sugars, then you will need to check the ingredient list. Flavored milks and flavored yogurts contain added sugars or sweeteners, so those will be out for this week.

- Vegetables of all types are great for this challenge. We encourage you to focus on green vegetables and leafy greens like broccoli, spinach, salad greens, and other vegetables like carrots, cucumbers, peas, cabbage, and cauliflower. Starchier vegetables like potatoes and corn are okay, but keep them to a minimum, ideally one or two servings per day at maximum.

- Whole grains get the green light. Look for grains that are high in fiber, like quinoa, farro, or brown or black rice as well as whole-grain options when possible for other carbohydrates like pasta, rice, crackers, and cereals. You can technically have refined grains as well, like white rice, regular pasta, and other wheat- and flour-based products, as they do not have added sugar, but they aren't the best choice because the body breaks them down quickly into glucose.

- Sources of protein like beans and legumes and proteins like meat, fish, and tofu are all recommended. Be careful when it comes to processed meats like bacon, sausage, hot dogs, salami, or other deli meats like honey ham or turkey, which often contain sugar (as well as preservatives).

Step 2: Get the Gang on Board

Success for your child will mean involving the whole family. Here's a good place to draw on some of the communication strategies from Chapter 6, "Sweet Talk: Motivate Your Family for Success."

Introduce the 7-Day Challenge to the adults in the house and ask for their support

Talk to your partner, stepparents, caregivers, and even to Grandma or Grandpa if they live with you or are involved with childcare activities. You should also talk to your co-parent if the kids will be in another household part of the week. Ideally, the whole family will be all in on this one. If you and your kids are going to cut out sugar for a week, it isn't going to work to have your partner there eating ice cream after dinner every night. You may be surprised that your kids adapt more easily than you do. Parents may also find they learn a lot about their own habits as they go along. As one of the dads who participated told us, "I used to think I ate really healthy, until I was on the fourth day and in need of a serious sugar fix! Now I'm much more cognizant of my sugar intake. I didn't think this challenge was going to have an impact on me. But it did."

Call a family meeting

If your kids are old enough to have a say in their food choices, you will need their buy-in. Choose a good time, when everyone is ready to talk, for a family meeting. If your kids are old enough to understand (around four years of age or older), get them as involved as much as possible. Older kids can read this chapter themselves to understand how the challenge works and can research recipes and even help prepare some of the new meals.

Here are some talking points you might find helpful:

- Express that you would like to challenge everyone, including yourself, to go one week without eating added sugar. If you pitch it like a challenge or even a dare, it becomes more fun. This isn't a diet, it's a nutrition challenge, and it's only for one week.

- Your kids may not understand why cutting sugar is important, so try to make it understandable and relevant to them. You can explain how it is hiding in lots of different foods and that too much of it isn't good for any of you. If you haven't already asked your kids to locate hidden sugar in your kitchen (page 30) or taken the Clif Bar Challenge (page 50), now is a good time. Kids hate to be tricked, so talk with them about how sugar marketing works, and ask them to imagine how much sugar they've been tricked into eating.

- Ask everyone what they think about the idea. Would they be willing to do it? What concerns do they have? Be sure to listen carefully to any reasons why your family is apprehensive.

- If your family doesn't seem at all willing to undertake this challenge, you have a few options. You can try the 28-Day Challenge instead. You can also shelve the idea for a few weeks and bring it up again later. You can also do the 7-Day Challenge yourself just to familiarize yourself with it. If your kids see you doing the challenge enthusiastically, they may decide to jump in or join you the next time around.

- Consider inviting friends or extended family to participate. With a larger group, you and your kids may find more motivation and more momentum for the challenge. The 7-Day Challenge can also be done as a group with other kids like youth groups, sports teams, or scout troops.

Reluctant Co-Parents

If you share your kids with their dad or mom part of the week, maybe you can get your co-parent's support—and maybe you can't. You may be able to complete the 7-Day Challenge in your home, only to send them off to another parent who has different views on sugar consumption, treats, and rewards. Try not to worry if this is the case. Even if the kids are exposed to more sugar than you would like in their co-parent's care, the exercise that you complete with your child in your own home can still have an impact on how they think about sugar. You might encounter some surprises: Your older kids, for example, may want to have a conversation with their other parent about health and changes they want to make. But ultimately, the 7-Day Challenge will teach them the importance of eating in a healthy way. They can eventually make smart choices regardless of household. If your child is not with you for seven days in a row, you can also consider doing the 28-Day Challenge instead, which does not require cutting out all sugar.

Involving Infants and Toddlers

If you have an infant or a young child who has started to eat solid food but isn't talking yet, you may wonder how the 7-Day Challenge will work. Although you don't need to secure the same kind of buy-in, you'll still need to be ready for objections. You know firsthand that kids this age can make their preferences known even without words! It helps to have something familiar to serve at each meal. They may be wondering where their favorite sweets have gone; by preparing a variety of non-sweetened foods they like, you'll increase the chances that your children will adapt and maybe even find some new foods they enjoy. If your toddler cries and asks for something sugary like juice, you can explain that you are not having juice today, and offer milk or water instead. Giving your child a choice of two healthy options allows for some autonomy. If your child is still feeling frustrated, try to change the mood by taking a walk, playing a game, or turning on some music.

Step 3: Get Everyone Motivated

Maybe your children have been complaining of being tired in class or not being able to run as fast as others at cross-country practice. Maybe your preteen is concerned about their skin. Or maybe your doctor has mentioned concern over your child's weight or identified signs of a metabolic issue like prediabetes that this challenge could begin to address. Each of these is a possible motivation for starting the 7-Day Challenge. And when you and your kids know their motivations, you'll all be more enthusiastic about the week ahead.

It's important to note that if your child is concerned about his or her weight, this can be a delicate and tricky subject to handle. We don't suggest doing this challenge as a means for losing weight. If possible, try to shift the focus away from weight to overall health and improved nutrition, as this challenge is not meant to be a weight-loss program or a diet.

In order to better understand each person's priorities, have each family member fill out the Motivation Tool below. You can assist younger children in filling out theirs. The first step is to list up to three benefits that might come about by doing this challenge. Then, in the next section of the form, each person will identify specific foods or drinks with added sugar that they will need to give up or replace for the week. Use the far-left column in the table below to make a list of some of the sweetened foods and drinks that you usually have. Examples include soda, juice, coconut water, granola bars, breakfast cereals, Gatorade, cookies, honey whole-wheat bread, ketchup, maple syrup, and coffee drinks. Write down the context of where and when you typically have these. Go through your list and think about how hard it will be to give these things up. Circle easy, medium, or hard for each. Go through and brainstorm some ideas of what you would be willing to have instead of each of the items on your list. Pay special attention to the ones that you think will be hard. Put a plan in a place that you feel good about.

Motivation Tool

Think about the reasons you want to do the 7-Day Challenge. How could you benefit from one week with no added sugar? List three benefits of your own. (If you are filling this out on behalf of a young child, you can list the benefits that you expect to see in your child.):

First Benefit: ....
Second Benefit: ....
Third Benefit: ....

Sweetened Foods or Drinks I Often Have and Where/When	How Easy Will It Be to Go without This? MARK 1 BOX			What Could I Have Instead? (TRY TO LIST THREE OPTIONS.)
	EASY	MEDIUM	HARD	
Example: Orange juice at breakfast		x		Tea or herbal tea; glass of milk; cut fruit
1.				
2.				
3.				
4.				
5.				
6.				
7.				

Sweetened Foods or Drinks I Often Have and Where/When	How Easy Will It Be to Go without This? MARK 1 BOX			What Could I Have Instead? (TRY TO LIST THREE OPTIONS.)
	EASY	MEDIUM	HARD	
8.				
9.				
10.				

Step 4: Pick Your Week

Next it's time to figure out when to do the challenge. Timing is important. Set yourself up for success by choosing a week where your family will be (mostly) together. If your kids will be away for a night or two with Grandma, who likes to offer the kids apple cobbler, it will be hard to succeed at this challenge. A week with out-of-town travel or too many school functions could be difficult, too. Decide the week with your challenge team and mark it on the calendar for everyone to see. We suggest starting on a Monday so you can use the weekend to do the planning and meal prep for the week.

Step 5: Check Everyday Staples for Hidden Sugars

Just for this week, you're going to avoid all foods with added sugar. Start by taking inventory of your kitchen and pantry. This means you'll need to read labels. Consult the lists of sugars and sweeteners on pages 29 and 53 so that you can identify any added sugar.

You might be surprised at what you find. We tapped two pediatric endocrinologists at Children's Hospital Los Angeles, Drs. Jennifer Raymond and Alaina Vidmar, to try an early version of the 7-Day Challenge with their families. Both have dedicated their careers to treating kids with obesity and diabetes, and they both have young kids. They know about the damaging effects that sugars can have on kids, and they thought they were doing their best to eat healthy, even with hectic schedules balancing work and family. And even these two clinical experts were shocked to discover how much sugar was lurking in their own pantries. Both said the same thing: "I didn't think there was that much sugar in our house, but we had to hunt for no-added-sugar items to replace many of our regular foods"; and "I also was so struck by how often products would say 'zero grams of added sugar' but then, when I checked the ingredients, they included items on the OUT list." These included products with things like stevia in them or processed foods with small amounts of added sugars like maltodextrin. So as you go through your kitchen, don't overlook these staples that may have added sugars or sweeteners:

○ Bread and bread products like whole grain bread or pizza dough
○ Crackers and other simple grain-based snacks
○ Breakfast cereals
○ Jarred sauces like pasta sauce or simmer sauces for meat
○ Dressings like salad dressing or mayo, including ranch dressings
○ Other condiments like ketchup, barbecue sauce, hot sauce, or pickle relish
○ Spreads like peanut butter, jelly, or jam. Watch for fruit spreads that say "all fruit" because they usually have fruit juice concentrate as an added sweetener.
○ Ready-made or frozen meals like frozen pizza
○ Breaded/battered meats like chicken nuggets and fish sticks
○ Processed meats like hot dogs, ham, bacon, sausage, honey-roasted turkey
○ Canned foods like baked beans and some soups (look for maltodextrin)
○ Spice mixes like taco seasoning
○ Commercially made smoothies and fruit drinks
○ Plant milks like vanilla soy or almond milk
○ Flavored yogurts and other milk-based products
○ Dried fruits that are sweetened such as cranberries or cherries and fruit strips

○ Granola bars and other healthy-sounding energy bars

○ Flavored, sweetened waters

○ Sports drinks, energy drinks, and sodas

○ Fruit-flavored or chocolate drink mixes

○ Jarred fruit sauces like applesauce

○ Premade pasta and rice mixes

You don't need to throw everything with added sugar away, but you need to be aware of what has added sugar—and it's best if you can move these items out of sight for now. Some families stash problematic canned goods in their emergency kits for earthquakes or other natural disasters.

Step 6: Create Your Personalized 7-Day Menu

The week will be much easier if you plan meals and snacks ahead of time. You can use our suggestions below to come up with a flexible plan that maximizes your family's buy-in. Many of the meals we suggest can be customized to meet individual needs because we know that each family and each kid is different.

Start by asking your family to help you create a list of possible breakfasts, lunches, dinners, and snacks that could work. Let everyone choose at least one breakfast, lunch, or dinner they'd like to see on the plan. That helps kids take ownership of the challenge and increases their willingness to participate. Get as much consensus as you can on meals, snacks, and beverages; then fill out a 7-Day Challenge Meal Plan (below) to keep track. You can use some of your usual favorites as a starting point and modify them as needed, or use our sample meal plans as a guide.

We want this plan to be easy for you, so you'll see that some of our recipes and meal suggestions work for breakfast, lunch, or dinner, allowing you to use leftovers interchangeably and save time. You can also use some convenience foods, like the ones we have suggested in the list below, but check the food labels and make sure they don't have added sugar. You can change things up as you go along, and repeats are just fine. If a particular item is a big hit, feel free to serve it again on another day.

Below are some suggestions, organized by meal, to get you started.

Breakfasts

SUGARPROOF RECIPES

- Egg in a Basket, page 281
- Popeye Scramble with Sweet Potato Toast, page 280
- Fuss-Free Frittata, page 279
- Overnight Steel-Cut Oats, Two Ways, page 292, or Overnight Chia Pudding Cups, page 294
- Three, Two, One... Crepes!, page 284
- Blueberry Banana Muffins, page 288
- Apple Plum Muffins, page 290
- "Fruit on the Top" Yogurt Pots, page 317
- Sugarproof Granola and Granola Thins, page 295
- Homemade Fennel Sausage Patties, page 282

OTHER CLASSIC OPTIONS

- Eggs Your Way (scrambled, fried, poached)
- Toast Your Way: top with avocado, smashed boiled egg, cheese, ricotta cheese, smoked salmon, hummus, or peanut/nut butter
- Plain yogurt with fruit and/or cereal (no added sugar, like Grape-Nuts)
- Plain oatmeal or other whole-grain porridge topped with nuts/seeds, fresh or dried fruits
- High-protein/high-fiber smoothie

Lunches

SUGARPROOF RECIPES

- Fuss-Free Frittata, page 279
- Three, Two, One... Crepes!, page 284
- "Fruit on the Top" Yogurt Pots, page 317
- One Big Soup, page 299
- Grilled Halloumi Salad, page 303

- Miso Soup with Tofu, page 305
- Roasted Vegetable Master Recipe, page 312
- Any of our snack recipes, see below

OTHER CLASSIC OPTIONS

- Sandwiches (plain or toasted) on bread with no added sugar (egg, cheese, turkey, tuna, etc.)
- Hummus and pita bread
- Cut-up raw vegetables
- Fresh fruit (like berries or grapes)
- Hard-boiled eggs
- Dinner leftovers
- Any snacks from the list below
- Tomato, mozzarella, basil on skewer

Dinners

SUGARPROOF RECIPES

- One Big Soup, page 299, with farro (or other whole grains)
- Loaded Veggie Chili, page 309
- Miso Soup with Tofu, page 305, with brown rice
- Grilled Halloumi Salad, page 303
- Broccoli and Sausage Pasta (Pasta Broccoli e Salsiccia), page 301
- Roasted Vegetable Master Recipe, page 312
- Homemade Fennel Sausage Patties, page 282
- Three, Two, One... Crepes!, page 284
- Tangerine Teriyaki Marinade/Sauce, page 337, with protein of choice
- Fuss-Free Frittata, page 279
- Turmeric Veggie Fried Rice, page 307

OTHER CLASSIC OPTIONS

- Grilled, baked, or pan-fried chicken, fish, or tofu
- Steamed, sautéed, or roasted vegetables

- Green or mixed salads with oil and vinegar (or other no-sugar added dressing)
- Whole-grain pasta
- Brown rice or other grain bowl meals
- Beans, lentils, or other legumes

Beverages

- Regular water
- Plain or sparkling water flavored with cucumber, citrus slices, berries or mint, or chunks/slices of other fresh or frozen fruit
- Store-bought sparkling water with natural flavoring (avoid those with artificial sweeteners)
- Milk or unsweetened nut/plant milk
- Tea or herbal tea (hot or iced)

Snacks

SUGARPROOF RECIPES

- Flax Thins Crackers, page 322
- Crispy Chickpea Snacks, page 316
- Tamari-Roasted Sunflower Seeds, page 318
- "Fruit on the Top" Yogurt Pots, page 317
- Roasted Red Cabbage Crisps, page 314
- Easy No-Bake Energy Bites, page 319
- Quick Carrot Cake Macaroons, page 321
- No-Bake Chocolate Sesame Squares, page 328
- Whole Fruit Pops, page 330
- Sugarproof Granola and Granola Thins, page 295

OTHER CLASSIC OPTIONS

- Edamame
- Seaweed snacks

○ Olives

○ Cheese

○ Raw veggies with or without dip

○ Fresh fruit

○ Sliced apple with nut butter

○ Nuts or seeds or popcorn

○ Plain yogurt

○ Whole-grain crackers with hummus or cream cheese

○ Toast topped with avocado, peanut butter, almond butter, cheese

○ Guacamole with vegetable slices or whole-grain chips

7-Day Challenge Meal Plan

	BREAKFAST	LUNCH	SNACKS	DINNER
Example Day: Thursday Date: Nov 1st	Sugarproof Granola with plain yogurt	Frittata squares, hummus, carrot sticks, whole-wheat pita bread	Curried Chickpea Snacks, sliced apple	Pasta with Sausage and Broccoli

Our 7-Day Challenge Meal Plan

	BREAKFAST	LUNCH	SNACKS	DINNER
Day 1 Day: Date:				
Day 2 Day: Date:				
Day 3 Day: Date:				

	BREAKFAST	LUNCH	SNACKS	DINNER
Day 4 Day: Date:				
Day 5 Day: Date:				
Day 6 Day: Date:				
Day 7 Day: Date:				

Beverage Options: List the beverages that you plan to have.
Example: Water flavored with cucumber slices

1. _____
2. _____
3. _____
4. _____
5. _____

A Sample Plan

This sample plan comes from a mom of three kids (ages four, seven, and ten) whose family performed the 7-Day Challenge. She truly made the plan her own. Instead of using the worksheet, she wrote out the plan in a way that made sense to her. (No matter whether you use the worksheet, it's important to write down your plan.) She mostly relied on recipes that she was already familiar with, though she did incorporate some of our Sugar-proof breakfast suggestions. Here's how her family worked the challenge:

BREAKFASTS

- Midweek days: Either a fried egg with a half avocado and/or toast, or toast with peanut butter.

- Weekend days: Three, Two, One . . . Crepes! (page 284) with sliced bananas sautéed in butter and some almond butter.

PACKED LUNCHES
- Havarti (or other cheese) and prosciutto sandwiches on sourdough bread or pita bread with hummus and veggies.
- Cucumber slices, cherry tomatoes, and cut fruit or tangerines.

DINNERS:
- Pork loin with apples and onions, served with jasmine rice
- Turkey meatball pitas
- Butternut squash chili
- Leftover pork loin with roasted potatoes and zucchini
- Split-pea soup with baguette
- Leftover meatballs with barley salad
- Tomatillo chicken soup

SNACKS:
- Raw vegetables (such as snap peas) and fruits; cucumber and hummus; banana or apple with peanut butter

You probably have family favorites you can incorporate into a plan like this—and now is a great time to try at least a couple of new recipes, such as those Three, Two, One . . . Crepes! (page 284), which this family enjoyed.

Step 7: Shop and Prep Wisely

We suggest that you shop in advance, so that you have almost everything in your house to make the meals and snacks you've planned. (You might need to make a few quick runs to the store later in the week for fresh proteins or produce.) Bring your kids along with you to pick out some of their own snacks and beverages, like a new box of herbal tea to drink hot or iced or their favorite fruits and vegetables.

The day before you start the challenge, use our ideas on pages 273–274 for advance prep. Invite your kids to help when possible. It can greatly increase their willingness to eat what is served.

Step 8: Monitor and Troubleshoot

At the end of each day, talk with your family about how it is going, and see if there have been any hiccups. Have everyone fill out the Evaluation Tool (below), which family members can use each day to reflect on how the challenge went and how they are feeling. You can help younger kids fill it in, or you can do it on their behalf, just to be aware of your child's mood and behavior.

Here are some of the common issues that come up during the 7-Day Challenge.

Eating out or ordering in

During the 7-Day Challenge, you may not be able to prepare all of your meals at home. If you end up at a restaurant or ordering in one night, you can still complete this challenge. Don't be afraid to ask questions when you order. Chain restaurants usually have nutrition information available, and perhaps even a list of ingredients, which will give you some clues. Smaller, independent restaurants may be making more things from scratch, so you can ask the waiter/cook/chef for more info about ingredients. As one of the moms who participated in the challenge told us, "My daughter and husband were dying to go to our favorite Mexican restaurant this week. I initially said no, but after much prompting I called the chef (whom we know because we frequent this restaurant) and he walked me through all of our favorite dishes. I was so surprised at how many no-sugar options there were on the menu."

Birthday parties or other social events

In a span of seven days, there's probably going to be a kid-specific event on the calendar. Yes, your children can still participate. You can talk with them about ways to keep the challenge on track, such as taking a Sugarproof treat to a birthday party to share or bringing a piece of cake home to save for next week. You may be surprised to realize after the challenge that the cake is not as important to your children as you might think.

School meals

It can be hard to know what exactly is in the food served for school breakfasts and lunches. If there is a menu available, you can help your children select options in advance, encouraging them to avoid flavored milk and juice as well as items with sweet sauces, like barbecue or teriyaki. You could talk with the cafeteria manager to find out more about ingredients, or you can skip school meals for the week and pack lunches instead. You may also want to consider if your children need any extra snacks or Sugarproof treats at school; if so, you can prepare and pack them in advance. Families report that their kids end up becoming their own advocates at school during the week of the challenge. Even one of the four-year-olds who participated told his nursery school teachers that he was having a "no-sugar family week." The news helped them modify the snacks they gave him.

Feeling awkward or embarrassed around other kids

It's normal for kids to want to fit in and have similar foods and drinks as their friends. Some kids, especially if they are shyer or more insecure, really don't like to stand out. Others are happy to be different and start new trends. You know your children best and can help them adjust. One great way to help is to pack extra snacks and encourage your kids to share with their friends and any other kids who are curious. This can work wonders to empower your kids and make them feel like cool trendsetters. Next thing you know, you'll be getting recipe requests from other parents in the class.

If your kids are still not comfortable with their new lunch options at school, modify the meal plan accordingly. This is supposed to be a challenge, not a punishment. If your child is not open to trying new foods, that is okay. You can still make the challenge work. There are plenty of classic options that don't have added sugar, like carrot sticks or string cheese, so don't worry if your child prefers to stick with what he or she already likes or what other kids are having at school.

Headaches

Headaches are a common symptom of sugar withdrawal, especially in the first few days. If your kids are used to caffeinated soft drinks, tea, coffee drinks, or energy drinks, any headaches this week could be caused by caffeine withdrawal as well. Staying hydrated usually helps a great deal. Sometimes a nap works wonders, too, because it addresses the fatigue that can come along with the headache. If time allows, you can suggest that your child lie down and rest. It's also helpful to avoid screen time when experiencing a headache. If the headache is really severe, and your child is older, you could offer some unsweetened black tea or green tea either hot or iced, to provide a small dose of caffeine, which will dilate the blood vessels and ease the headache.

Lethargy or irritability

Both are normal to be expected with a sudden elimination of sugar, so be prepared. Remember, sugar is addictive. If your children are used to a regular sugar fix, they may become quite grumpy when they don't get it. Fatigue and bad moods should subside within a few days. Try easing the sugar withdrawals by drinking extra water and having fresh fruit available. As one of our participating moms explained to her children, "You are feeling bad right now because you are used to having processed food and sugar, and your body is upset. You can try some sugar in a natural form, like fruit."

Hunger

If some of your kid's favorite snack foods are off the menu for this week, they may feel at a loss for what to eat, or they may refuse to eat something new that you offer. Be sure to have extra snacks on hand, ones that you know they like and that don't have added sugar.

Step 9: Evaluate Next Steps

After you have completed the 7-Day Challenge, talk with your family about their experiences and ask how they are feeling after the week. To help you structure the conversation, we've created several worksheets for you: an Evaluation Tool; Positives, Negatives, and Notes; and a Post-Challenge Recap. You'll find these worksheets at the end of this chapter. The input from this family debriefing is vital. You'll use this information to help your family members identify the ways they feel different without sugar, and you can spot the changes your family can sustain for the long term.

Be sure to congratulate yourself—and your entire family—for accepting the challenge and taking the plunge. You've just accomplished something you and your kids should be very proud of. Even if they weren't always enthusiastic about the experience, praise them for what they did do well.

Even improving one or two sugar-related habits is a major feat. Several of the parents we have worked with agree and shared their victories with us. One said, "I am already calling this experiment a success because my kid successfully switched to a no-sugar brand of peanut butter without problems and has not looked back." Another mom was able to wean her daughter off of store-bought juice and smoothies. "I think we have broken our juice habit. That in itself is huge. Before, I would try to limit it to one cup a day and try to water it down. Now I offer them a banana or some apple slices instead. My daughter was upset at first, at least for the first few times I said no, but then she accepted it. Instead I proposed unsweetened rooibos tea, which is something that the kids like from Starbucks, and now I make it at home."

Moving Forward

Before you think about moving forward, you should first consider what *not* to do. Don't ruin all your hard work by immediately bingeing on sugar with your family. It might be tempting to celebrate by taking the kids out for ice cream or doughnuts, but you don't want to undo the great start you have made. You have likely already seen the positive changes in mood and have successfully reset your taste buds to be more sensitive to sugar. You will notice that after the one-week washout period, kids are happier with less sugar and more receptive to new offerings.

Make the most of this important juncture in your family's eating habits. Instead of going right back to where you used to be, you can:

- Continue on for another week, or even longer. Some families find they are doing so well with the challenge that they want to extend it two or three weeks, or even a full month of no added sugar. For some families, the initial week is only the start, and once they get the hang of it and work through the cravings, it becomes easier. They want to keep going.

- Agree on some long-term changes that reduce sugar. You may discover that some of the new foods your family ate during the challenge are ones they want to keep having. Perhaps you found a new bread that you like, or a new breakfast that doesn't revolve around cereal and juice.

- Be thoughtful about what you let back into your house. As a mother told us, "Now we let less sugar in the house. I just stop it earlier, at the store, instead of trying to fight the battle after it has already come into the house." She and other parents have realized that their home should ideally be a low-sugar refuge.

- Come back to the challenge again when you need it. This challenge can be repeated monthly, yearly, or whenever you think your family could use a reset with sugar. Keep track of what worked and the benefits your family enjoyed so you can build on your progress each time you try it again.

We don't expect that you'll continue on indefinitely with no added sugar. We know that in most situations, it's just not realistic. But with the challenge under your belt, it's smart to identify some new strategies. Valentina told us, "My question to myself going forward is, 'What's worth the added sugar'?" And Gina said, "Moving forward, I will be more cognizant of where the sugars are, and of choosing the lower-sugar option. But I won't worry about birthday parties. They need to have their childhood. It's all about the balance." We couldn't have said it better. Sugarproofing for the long term isn't about angry deprivation; it's about moderation. By spending just one week without sugar, you can help guide your family to its own best, healthiest path.

Evaluation Tool: Record Your Experience

Use this evaluation to record how you are feeling each day as you go through the 7-Day Challenge and to discuss how it went. Each member of the family can complete their own self-evaluation. Younger kids will need some help filling this in. You may see that the amount of sugar you crave goes down over the week and that you have more energy. But it is okay and normal if you have some ups and downs. You may also see that you start to like the low-sugar foods and drinks more as you get used to them.

DATE:	DAY 1	DAY 2	DAY 3	DAY 4	DAY 5	DAY 6	DAY 7
How much did you crave sugar today? PUT AN X IN ONE BOX FOR EACH DAY							
A lot							
Some							
Not much							
Not at all							

DATE:	DAY 1	DAY 2	DAY 3	DAY 4	DAY 5	DAY 6	DAY 7
How much energy did you have today? PUT AN X IN ONE BOX FOR EACH DAY							
A lot							
Some							
Not much							
Not at all							
How much did you like what you ate and drank today? PUT AN X IN ONE BOX FOR EACH DAY							
A lot							
Some							
Not much							
Not at all							

Positives, Negatives, and Notes

Use this space to write down things that went well and things that didn't go well each day, or any positive or negative experiences. For example, if you enjoyed having fruit for dessert, write that as a positive, or if you really missed ice cream, write that in the negative side. Feel free to add in any other notes about your day.

LIST SOME OF YOUR EXPERIENCES FOR EACH DAY:			
	POSITIVE (IF ANY)	NEGATIVE (IF ANY)	NOTES
Example	*I was able to avoid drinking soda*	*I had a headache and was in a bad mood*	*My head felt better after I had some water*
Day 1			
Day 2			
Day 3			

LIST SOME OF YOUR EXPERIENCES FOR EACH DAY:			
	POSITIVE (IF ANY)	NEGATIVE (IF ANY)	NOTES
Day 4			
Day 5			
Day 6			
Day 7			

Post-Challenge Recap
Graph Your Progress

At the end of the week, go back to the first page of this evaluation tool and graph your progress by drawing a line to connect the seven boxes that you marked for the days of the week. For example, your graph for sugar cravings might look like this (see below). In this case, cravings for sugar went down over the week. What happened with your cravings and energy levels? And did you start to like the food and beverages more?

DATE:	DAY 1	DAY 2	DAY 3	DAY 4	DAY 5	DAY 6	DAY 7
How much did you crave sugar today? PUT AN X IN ONE BOX FOR EACH DAY							
A lot	x	x					
Some			x	x			
Not much					x	x	
Not at all							x

Questions to Discuss with Your Family

1. How did it feel to undertake this challenge? As the week went on, did you start to have more positive experiences? Did you have

more energy? Were you happier? How was your mood? Could you concentrate better in class?

2. What worked well for your family during this challenge? What (if anything) didn't work as well? What were the easiest things to go without and what were the hardest?

3. Did anything surprise you about the experience?

4. Did you try any new staple foods (basic foods that you eat every day)? If so, list them here:

_____

_____

_____

_____

Would any of these work as permanent replacements for what you used to buy? For example, could you continue buying bread with no added sugar, or sparkling water rather than soda?

5. Did you try out any new recipes with no added sugar? If so, list them here:

_____

_____

_____

What did your family think of them? Would you be willing to have them again?

6. Did you try any new snacks? If so, list them here:

_____

_____

_____

_____

Would you be willing to have any of these regularly?

7. What did you learn from doing this challenge?

8. Now that the challenge is over, which of your successes would be the easiest to keep up with? Some of these may be things you noted in questions #4 to #6 above. Are there any things you would like to compromise on? Oftentimes there is a happy middle ground. If you do decide to add sugar back in, could you add less? For example, were your kids used to ordering sweetened iced tea from a local cafe? Instead of ordering the standard amount of sweetener that comes by default, could they ask for just 1 pump of sugar? Or ask for no sugar and put only a ½ packet in themselves?

Notes for the future: If you were to do this challenge again, is there anything you would do differently?

To view the scientific references cited in this chapter, please visit us online at sugarproofkids.com/bibliography.

CHAPTER NINE

The 28-Day Challenge: A Gradual Plan for Rightsizing Sugar

When the 7-Day Challenge works, it really works. But for some families—and you know who you are—it's simply unrealistic. That's perfectly fine. For you, a more gradual reduction in sugar is the key to Sugarproof success. Sometimes it isn't how quickly you cut the sugar—what matters is that you *do* cut the sugar. The 28-Day Challenge will help you ease into the changes.

With this plan, we'll help you take stock of your family's diet, identify high-sugar culprits, and gradually reduce sugar. You'll learn some hacks and makeovers that will help you upgrade your family's food and beverage repertoire, depend less on added sugars, and get closer to the recommended sugar intake for healthy growth.

How do you know if the gradual approach is best for you and your family?

Do you have a picky eater? Many parents choose the 28-Day Challenge because they have children who are in an especially picky phase with their eating habits. Taking away their "safe" foods and suddenly replacing them with other options might not go so well. With the gradual plan, you can set small goals, such as reducing how often you serve highly processed granola bars and crackers for snacks.

Are you afraid of a backlash? A gradual approach might work better if you have a child (or adult) who seems to have become addicted to a sweet diet. Taking away sweet drinks and other foods might cause too much disruption in the house or trigger a backlash of overeating. With the 28-Day Challenge, you can create a slower plan to break your kids' addictions to soda, sweetened yogurts, fruit snacks, sugary cereal, and nightly desserts more gradually.

Does your family have a hard-to-break nightly dessert habit? If mealtimes have become a battle over sweet treats, a gradual approach might reduce the fighting. Instead of cutting the nightly ice cream, cookies, and candy, a slower change will help you introduce alternatives or cut dessert down to just one or two nights a week.

Is your family's schedule jam-packed with activities? Take a look at the family calendar to see how busy everyone is in the upcoming weeks. If you're all busy with classes, practice, and lessons or summer camp and swim meets, the 28-Day Challenge might be a better fit—for you and for them. With this gradual plan, you can allow for days that include added sugar.

Some additional ways that the 28-Day Challenge is different from the 7-Day Challenge:

- It doesn't require you to put away the sugary foods you currently have on hand, as we suggest in the 7-Day Challenge. You can use up what's in your refrigerator and pantry, even if it has some added sugar in it, before you work on gradually eliminating these items from your diet.
- There are no strict guidelines. You can go about slowly reducing sugar on your own terms, or you can address just one source of added sugar at a time, which can be less overwhelming for some families than trying to work on everything at once. It's all up to you and what works best for your family.

- For families in which not everyone is fully on board, we offer a stealth option, carried out by whoever is responsible for the household shopping and meal prep. Busy teens or very young children might not even notice—or care enough to put up a fuss— but you will notice the results.

If you're preparing most of the meals, you're the expert on what everyone in the family likes to eat. You also have inside knowledge about the sugary culprits in your family's food choices. With the 28-Day Challenge, you can gather ideas to create your own plan based on family preferences. Each family will have a different starting point and likely different end goals as well. No matter which options you choose, an important part of this plan is weaning your kids and family off the sugary staples they are used to.

The 28-Day Challenge, Step by Step

The 28-Day Challenge includes six steps. Because this approach is less drastic than the 7-Day Challenge, you have more flexibility in some of these areas.

- Decide on Your Approach: Family or Stealth?
- Identify the Usual Culprits
- Choose Your Goals
- Plot Your Steps
- Track Your Progress
- Conclude and Reflect

Step 1: Decide on Your Approach: Family or Stealth?

When it comes to tackling this challenge, you've got two options. Drop a few hints to your family about cutting back on sugar and gauge the response. Depending on what you hear, you may want to approach the 28-Day Challenge collectively as a family—or go "stealth."

The Family Approach

If everyone seems ready to try cutting back on sugar, choose a time to sit down together and come up with a game plan. Getting kids involved in the planning can be instrumental in their willingness to participate and the overall success of the challenge. Don't underestimate the ability of young children to grasp the idea of reducing sugar. One family with two small children was surprised when their kids explained that they needed to cut back on sugar "because we want to live a long time and be healthy."

Find Your Sweet Spot

A fun way to kick off a family challenge is to determine everyone's Sugarproof Sweet Spot at your initial family meeting (see page 251). The Sugarproof Sweet Spot test involves each family member tasting versions of sweetened drinks like juice or sweetened staples like yogurt with different amounts of sugar in them. You can then rate your sweet taste preferences at the start of the four weeks. Repeat the test again at the end of the month to see if anyone's "sweet spot" has shifted toward less sweetness.

Go Stealth

Maybe your kids are too young to understand. Maybe your kids or partner are just not buying into the idea. If you would rather skip potential conflict, you can work on some changes yourself that will benefit the family. If you're in control of the grocery shopping and food prep, you're in a unique position to make subtle changes on your own over the course of the month. Your family might not notice all the changes, but you'll notice the health benefits.

There are a variety of ways to go stealth. You can skip store-bought, premade cookies and use a Sugarproof recipe to make some alternative treats. You can dilute orange juice with water to reduce its sweetness. You could even skip buying juice at all for a week or two. Instead, you could purchase whole oranges and slice them to put on the breakfast table instead of the juice. Yes, it's a little sneaky, but it may be what works best. Ultimately, what you buy and serve is up to you.

Step 2: Identify the Usual Culprits

What are the sweet items your family eats or drinks on a regular basis? These might be the energy bars your eight-year-old loves, or your partner's daily can of diet soda—and they're what we call the Usual Culprits. They're probably some of the biggest sources of sugar or sweeteners in your family's diet. To succeed at the 28-Day Challenge, you won't need to get rid of all of your family's Usual Culprits, but you definitely need to know what they are. That way, you can decide which ones you want to tackle. We've identified some of the most common Culprits below.

Usual Culprits, Breakfast Items

- Sweetened cereal or oatmeal
- Sweetened yogurts
- Granola/breakfast bars
- Toast with jam
- Pancakes or waffles with syrup
- Pastries/muffins
- Juices (or smoothies that contain juice)

Usual Culprits, Beverages

- Soda
- Diet sodas or other diet drinks
- Sports drinks
- Energy drinks

- Sweetened teas, coffees, and Frappuccinos
- Juice and juice drinks (includes 100 percent juice)
- Coconut water
- Vitamin Water and other sweetened waters
- Commercially made smoothies
- Flavored milks

Usual Culprits, Snacks and Lunch Box Items

- Granola bars
- Sweetened yogurts
- Fruit snacks or rolls
- Juice boxes
- Cookies/graham crackers
- Trail mixes with candy and/or sweetened dried fruits like cranberries
- Spreads that have added sugars, such as many peanut butters
- Jelly or jam (even if it says "all fruit" or "sugar free")
- Breads and lunch meats (most have some added sugar)
- Candy
- Pudding or Jell-O cups

Usual Culprits, Dinners

- Teriyaki sauces
- Pasta with jarred sauce that contains added sugars
- Barbecue sauce or ketchup
- Salad dressings and other condiments
- Frozen meals/breaded meats like chicken nuggets and fish sticks
- Baked beans
- Canned soups
- Spice mixes, such as taco seasoning

Usual Culprits, Treats and Desserts

○ Candies

○ Chocolates

○ Ice cream and other frozen treats

○ Pies, cakes, cookies, brownies, etc.

To identify your family's Usual Culprits, take some time to fill in the worksheet we've made for you. To make sure you aren't forgetting anything, take a look through your refrigerator and pantry. If your family is participating, each person can make their own. Once your kids make their lists, you might get a surprise or two. Remind them that everything counts, including whatever they buy at coffee shops, order in restaurants, or eat at school. (You can find the grams of sugar per serving on the labels for foods in your pantry or online for chain restaurants and coffee shops. Don't forget to check the portion sizes against what you eat or drink. Those sugar grams can add up fast.) If you're taking the stealth approach, map out Culprits that you know your family is consuming. You might not know what is happening outside the home, and that's okay for now.

After you make your list, tally up the sugars. Your long-term goal is to bring sugar down to our recommended daily amount. To make things easier, we've created a chart, "Your Family's Sugar Guidelines," that lets you fill in each family member's daily sugar recommendation; consult page 66 in Chapter 2 to find this information. Your final tally of sugars won't be a perfect estimate, because some of the labels will include sugar that is naturally occurring (not added), such as the lactose in yogurt or milk. Nevertheless, you'll have a good idea of how close you are to the guidelines.

A note about measurements: Food labels, as well as the daily recommendations, measure sugar in grams. But we want you to convert the total grams to teaspoons, as a way of wrapping your head around just how much sugar your family is consuming. To convert grams to teaspoons, just divide the number of grams by four.

Usual Culprits for:_____
(Complete one per family member)

Category	Item	Type of Added Sugar	Approximate Total Sugar per Serving	Approximate Times per Week Eating	Total Sugar per Week from This Item
Breakfasts					
Beverages					
Snacks/ Lunch Box Items					
Dinner					
Treats and Desserts					
TOTAL SUGAR					___g sugar/week ___g sugar/day ___tsp sugar/day (To caluculate the tsp of sugar per day, divide the grams by 4)

Sample Usual Culprits (for a Thirteen-Year-Old Boy):

Category	Item	Type of Added Sugar	Approximate Total Sugar per Serving	Approximate Times per Week Eating	Total Sugar per Week from This Item
Breakfasts	Rice Krispies	Sugar (sucrose)	4g per 1¼ cups	3	12g
	Krusteaz Original Pancakes with ¼ cup maple syrup	Sugar (sucrose) and maple syrup	5g per ⅓ cup (makes three 4" pancakes) plus 47g for the syrup = 52g	1	52g
	Toast with strawberry jam (Oroweat Organic 22 Grains & Seeds Bread, Non-GMO and Smucker's Strawberry Jam)	Cane sugar, high-fructose corn syrup, corn syrup, sugar	4g per slice for the bread plus 12g of sugar for 1 tbs of jam = 16g	3	48g
	Chocolate milk (Horizon Organic Box)	Organic cane sugar	22g per 8FO box	5	110g
Beverages	Dr Pepper	High-fructose corn syrup	40g per 12-oz. can	3	120g
	Vitamin Water Zero Power C Dragonfruit	erythritol, stevia leaf extract	0g	3	0g
	Tropicana Orange Juice 100% plus calcium (no pulp)	Fruit juice (mixed composition of sugars)	22g per 8FO	4	88g
	Tea with honey or sugar (made at home)	Honey or sugar	2 tsp (8g) per mug	3	24g

Category	Item	Type of Added Sugar	Approximate Total Sugar per Serving	Approximate Times per Week Eating	Total Sugar per Week from This Item
Snacks/ Lunch Box Items	Teddy Grahams Snack Pack	Sugar, dextrose, honey, malto-dextrose	7g per pack	4	28g
	Nature Valley Oats and Honey Crunchy Granola Bars	Sugar, honey, brown sugar syrup	11g per 2 bars (1 pack)	4	44g
	Yoplait Original Strawberry Kiwi Yogurt	Sugar	19g	5	95g
	Welch's Fruit Snacks Mixed Fruit	Corn syrup, sugar, grape juice from concentrate	11g per pouch	5	55g
	Oroweat Organic 22 Grains & Seeds Bread, non-GMO	Cane sugar	4g per slice	7	28g
Dinner	Prego Traditional Pasta Sauce	Sugar	9g per ½ cup	1	9g
	Teriyaki Chicken (Yoshinoya Regular Bowl)	Sugar	16g	1	16g
	California roll sushi (Genji brand)	Sugar	14g in one 6-piece roll	1	14g

Category	Item	Type of Added Sugar	Approximate Total Sugar per Serving	Approximate Times per Week Eating	Total Sugar per Week from This Item
Treats and Desserts	Swedish fish	Sugar, invert sugar, corn syrup	31g in 7 pieces	2	62g
	Breyers Chocolate Mint Ice Cream	Sugar, corn syrup	16g in ½ cup	2	32g
	Oreo Cookies	Sugar, high-fructose corn syrup	14g in 3 cookies	2	28g
	Chocolate Brownie	Sugar	33g in a 4" square	1	33g
TOTAL SUGAR					898g sugar per week 128g sugar per day 32 tsp sugar per day

Your Family's Sugar Guidelines

Use the table on page 66 to create easy-to-read sugar guidelines for each member of the family and keep this information handy:

FAMILY MEMBER NAME AND AGE

SUGARPROOF MAXIMUM DAILY SUGAR RECOMMENDATION

g/day tsp/day

g/day tsp/day

g/day tsp/day

g/day tsp/day

g/day tsp/day

Step 3: Choose Your Goals

The Usual Culprits tell you what the biggest contributors to your family's sugar consumption are. Use this information to identify up to four specific goals for the 28-Day Challenge. It can be helpful to create goals around categories, such as breakfast or beverages.

These goals can be for the whole family or specific members. If you're going stealth, focus on what you can control. For the family approach, either decide to set goals as a family, or let everyone set their own goals. We'll start you off with some suggestions, broken down by category.

IDEAS FOR BREAKFAST GOALS

- Replace highly sweetened cereals with less sweetened versions.
- Replace juice with whole or cut fresh fruit.
- Add sources of protein and fiber.
- Replace traditional baked goods like muffins with alternatives from our Sugarproof recipes.
- Try some new breakfast ideas on a few mornings per week such as Fuss-Free Frittata (page 279), Popeye Scramble with Sweet Potato Toast (page 280), Overnight Steel-Cut Oats, Two Ways (page 292), Blueberry Banana Muffins (page 288), Apple Plum Muffins (page 290), or Three, Two, One . . . Crepes! (page 284).

IDEAS FOR BEVERAGE GOALS

- Order fewer sodas when out and limit the quantity by not getting refills and by ordering with more ice.
- Order lower-sugar drink alternatives at coffee shops by requesting 75 percent, 50 percent, and eventually 25 percent sweetness.
- Replace juice with whole fruit.
- Start drinking water with meals, making it the default choice.
- Invest in a water filter and/or bottles to store in the fridge, making it easy to reach for when thirsty and to put on the table at mealtimes.

IDEAS FOR LUNCH/SNACK GOALS

- Replace peanut butter and jelly sandwiches with plain unsweetened peanut butter or peanut butter and banana (or another type of sandwich altogether).
- Make Sugarproof snacks like granola thins (see Sugarproof Granola and Granola Thins, page 295), Crispy Chickpea Snacks (page 316), or Easy No-Bake Energy Bites (page 319) to use in the lunch box and for after-school snacks.
- Find different options at the store that don't contain added sugar such as nuts, seeds, cheeses, or bars with no added sugar and sweetened with dried fruit.

IDEAS FOR DINNER GOALS

- Plan meals and cook more often at home to avoid sugar when eating out.
- Replace commercially bought sauces, such as pasta sauce, with zero-added-sugar options (homemade or store-bought); see recipe for our Basic Sugarproof Pasta and Pizza Sauce on page 336.
- Add more vegetables to replace the foods you want to eat less of. Increasing vegetables at meals will displace other less healthy options.

IDEAS FOR TREATS/DESSERT GOALS

- Reduce the frequency of desserts to once or twice a week.
- Reduce portion size and serve on smaller plates.
- Limit candy to weekends only.
- Eat healthier candy alternatives, such as nuts or dried, unsweetened fruit.

Which changes appeal most to you and your family? List your goals in the space we've provided. Try to keep things simple and achievable. When possible, make them measurable as well. If you're cutting back on sugary after-school snacks, measure by the portion or the number of days in the week you have them. If you're trying to cut back on juice, measure by the ounces before you dilute them or the number of glasses in the morning. For inspiration, take a look at the goals for the thirteen-year-old boy who filled out the Usual Culprits worksheet (page 236). He'd been consuming around 128 grams, or 32 teaspoons, of sugar each day. That's roughly five times our maximum recommended amount for his age. To gradually reduce his sugar intake, he could work on four goals simultaneously choosing from the following ideas:

Goal 1—Breakfast: Gradually replace chocolate milk with regular milk (or Sugarproof Homemade Chocolate Milk, page 334); gradually replace sugary cereals with other non-sugar or negligible sugar options; gradually cut down on the jam and maple syrup used for toast and pancakes, having them only on one weekend day and replacing them with nut butter or sliced banana for weekdays.

Goal 2—Beverages: Gradually dilute apple or orange juice and eventually substitute with plain water and/or apple and orange slices or other fresh fruit; replace the Dr Pepper with other flavored non-sweetened beverages.

Goal 3—Lunches/Snacks: Exchange prepackaged items like Teddy Grahams and fruit snacks for easy homemade options like trail mix and Easy No-Bake Energy Bites (page 319).

Goal 4—Treats/Desserts: Gradually reduce Swedish fish from twice a week to once a month and replace with any of our Sugarproof treats, such as Whole Fruit Pops (page 330) or No-Bake Chocolate Sesame Squares (page 328).

By focusing on some of the biggest sources of sugar, you can make a big dent in cutting down on average daily sugar intake. If this boy could gradually remove the chocolate milk, orange juice, Dr Pepper, fruit snacks, and Swedish fish, his average total daily sugar intake would be cut in half—from 128 grams (32 teaspoons) to 64 grams (16 teaspoons). That saves around 112 teaspoons of sugar each week. He would still be over the daily maximum, but he'd have taken a big step in the right direction. For this extreme sugar consumer, we would recommend repeated 28-Day Challenges to gradually work toward the recommended amount.

By the end of the 28-Day Challenge, your family will have begun to take control over added sugars and sweeteners. This doesn't mean you'll have a diet that is totally free of sugar. The goal is to keep it close to the recommended amounts, with no LCS. If there are multiple issues to work on and four weeks is not long enough to address all of the Usual Culprits, you can always do another round of the challenge at a later date.

GOALS FOR THE 28-DAY CHALLENGE
List up to four goals. You can complete one list per _person_ or one list per _family_:

1. _____
2. _____
3. _____
4. _____

Step 4: Plot Your Steps

Now that you have listed your goals, you have two options for easing into change. You can gradually work toward your goals over the month, or you can work on one goal each week. Decide which you prefer. If you are doing the family approach, try letting your kids decide which option they like best.

Option 1: Slow and Steady: Gradually Work toward Your Goals

At the outset of the plan, don't ask your kids to give up their favorite sweet item. Instead, have them reduce that item a little more each week. If it's a drink, dilute it. If it's food, slowly replace it. Here are some examples.

USUAL CULPRIT BEFORE CHALLENGE	WEEK 1 1st Step	WEEK 2 2nd Step	WEEK 3 3rd Step	WEEK 4 Arrive at Goal
Target area: Breakfasts				
Chocolate milk	¾ chocolate milk mixed with ¼ plain milk	½ chocolate milk mixed with ½ plain milk	¼ chocolate milk mixed with ¾ plain milk (OR Sugarproof Homemade Chocolate Milk)	Plain milk (OR Sugarproof Homemade Chocolate Milk)
Toast and jam	Toast with less jam	Toast with even less jam and the addition of peanut butter or nut butter	Toast with nut or peanut butter and banana slices or raisins	Toast with another protein and/or healthy fat, e.g., soft cheese such as ricotta or sliced hard cheese, avocado, peanut or nut butter
High-sugar cereal	¾ high-sugar cereal mixed with ¼ plain cereal of choice	½ sweetened and ½ plain cereal	¼ sweetened and ¾ plain cereal topped with fresh fruit (optional)	Unsweetened cereal topped with fresh fruit (optional)
Fruit juice at breakfast	¾ cup juice, ¼ cup water	½ cup juice, ½ cup water	¼ cup juice, ¾ cup water	Water or unsweetened herbal tea
Target area: Lunches				
Peanut butter and jelly sandwich	Peanut butter and jelly sandwich with less jelly	Peanut butter sandwich with thin banana slices	Plain peanut butter sandwich	Other sandwich of choice for variety: avocado and cheese, tuna, turkey, etc.
3 Oreo cookies	2 Oreo cookies	1 Oreo cookie plus one Sugarproof No-Baked Chocolate Sesame Square	2 Sugarproof No-Bake Chocolate Sesame Squares or Easy No-Bake Energy Bites	1 Sugarproof No-Bake Chocolate Sesame Square or Easy No-Bake Energy Bite

USUAL CULPRIT BEFORE CHALLENGE	WEEK 1 1st Step	WEEK 2 2nd Step	WEEK 3 3rd Step	WEEK 4 Arrive at Goal
Target area: Lunches				
Capri Sun pouch undiluted	Water bottle with ¾ Capri Sun, ¼ water	Water bottle with ½ Capri Sun, ½ water	Water bottle with ¼ Capri Sun, ¾ water	Water bottle with just water
Target area: Dinners				
Pasta with jarred sauce that contains added sugar	Pasta with jarred sauce mixed with Italian tomato passata (3 to 1 ratio) or store-bought sauce without added sugar	Pasta with jarred sauce mixed with Italian tomato passata (1 to 1 ratio) or unsweetened sauce of choice	Pasta with jarred sauce mixed with Italian tomato passata (1 to 3 ratio) or other unsweetened sauce	Basic Sugarproof Pasta and Pizza Sauce made with Italian tomato passata (see recipe), or store-bought sauce with no added sugar
Teriyaki chicken	Teriyaki chicken with 75% of the sauce	Teriyaki chicken with ½ of the sauce	Teriyaki chicken with ¼ of the sauce	Chicken with Sugarproof Tangerine Teriyaki Marinade/ Sauce (or other marinade/ seasonings with no added sugar)
Fast-food meal with a soda	Fast-food meal with ¾ of a soda (can either decrease portion or dilute with club soda)	Fast-food meal with ½ of a soda (can either decrease portion or dilute with club soda)	Fast-food meal with ¼ of a soda (can either decrease portion or dilute with club soda)	Fast-food meal with club soda (or sparkling water) with lemon or lime (optional) or plain water
Target area: Snacks				
Gummy fruit snacks or Sour Patch Kids (1 package)	¾ package, ½ cup fresh berries or grapes	½ package, ¾ cup berries or grapes	¼ package, ¾ cup berries or grapes and a handful of nuts	1 cup berries or grapes and a handful of nuts

USUAL CULPRIT BEFORE CHALLENGE	WEEK 1 1st Step	WEEK 2 2nd Step	WEEK 3 3rd Step	WEEK 4 Arrive at Goal
Target area: Snacks				
Granola bars	¾ granola bar, ¼ cup homemade trail mix (no added sugar)	½ granola bar, ⅓ cup homemade trail mix	¼ granola bar with ½ cup homemade trail mix	¾ cup homemade trail mix or Sugarproof Granola Thins
Fruit-flavored yogurt	¾ cup fruit-flavored yogurt mixed with ¼ cup plain yogurt	½ cup fruit-flavored yogurt mixed with ½ cup plain yogurt	¼ cup fruit-flavored yogurt mixed with ¾ cup plain yogurt and fresh fruit	1 cup plain yogurt topped with sliced fresh fruit or berries
Target area: Desserts				
Every night	Every other night	Every third night	Every fourth night	Once a week
Full portion	¾ portion	½ portion	¼ portion	Sugarproof dessert (see recipe ideas)

Option 2: Knock Out One Goal per Week

Or you can work on one goal at time, building on each week like this:

	WEEK 1	WEEK 2	WEEK 3	WEEK 4
Goal 1	**Make Change**	Maintain Change	Maintain Change	Maintain Change
Goal 2	Usual Habits	**Make Change**	Maintain Change	Maintain Change
Goal 3	Usual Habits	Usual Habits	**Make Change**	Maintain Change
Goal 4	Usual Habits	Usual Habits	Usual Habits	**Make Change**

Leslie, a mom from Oregon, worked with her family with this progressive approach. She and her husband talked to their kids, who were ages twelve and nine, about what they were doing and why. Together, the family decided on four goals—and they wanted to work on one each week. By the end of the 28-Day Challenge, they had cut sugar out of all four categories. Here are Leslie's notes on how her family's plan took shape:

Week 1 (Breakfast): Switched from their favorite maple brown sugar oatmeal to a homemade low-sugar version. Switched cereal from Reese's Puffs and Frosted Mini-Wheats to plain Cheerios and Kix.

Week 2 (Beverages): Cut out all juice and soda and replaced with Arrowhead brand sparkling water. Gradually depleted the Usual Culprits from the pantry. As Leslie noted, "We were drinking Sparkling Ice (which seemed sugar free until I looked at the label and realized there was sucralose in it) and occasionally we would let them have a mini can of Sprite or Coke or some apple juice. Once we ran out of those drinks, we just didn't buy them anymore."

Week 3 (Snacks/lunch box items): Replaced granola bars and fruit snacks with fruit and nuts.

Week 4 (Treats and Desserts): Limited the number of nights that the kids could have dessert, allowing it only on the weekends.

Step 5: Track Your Progress

As you go through the four weeks of the challenge, take time each week to note how it is going. Ask your kids how they're feeling about the challenge, and keep track of how you and the other adults in the household are sticking to the plan. If you're using the stealth approach, ask yourself whether anyone has noticed that you're cutting back on portion sizes or not buying their favorite soda. Use the Weekly Reflection Tool to record your thoughts and observations as well as new ideas for reducing sugar. If you're following the family approach, older children and other family members can keep their own notes or diary.

Step 6: Conclude and Reflect

To conclude the challenge and measure your progress, try the Family Experiment again to see how your tastes have changed. After four weeks of gradually reducing sugar, chances are your family will like more diluted beverages or less sweetened foods. Their bliss point, or taste for sweetness, has changed—and your children are not only eating less sugar, they crave it less.

Has your family formed any new habits? They may point out that for the first two weeks they had to think about what they were eating, but by the end, they'd made conscious choices to replace old favorites with low-sugar options. Or you may find that new habits you've created during the 28-Day Challenge have led to permanent changes for your family. How many of your Usual Culprits have you been able to eat or drink less frequently or cut out entirely?

Once your family has adjusted to a lower-sugar diet, the next step is to maintain it. Families we have worked with have found it natural to continue with many of the changes they made, likely because they gradually eased into them. And because they experienced improvements in mood and energy levels, they felt motivated to continue on. What's more, the kids who actively participated became advocates in their own houses, even advising their own parents on Sugarproof choices.

Here are some testimonials from parents who completed the 28-Day Challenge:

"We will continue with all of the changes because although the changes were small, the kids are sleeping better and feeling better. They seem to have more energy and don't 'crash' as hard at the end of the day. Honestly, they were really open to all the changes. I think because they are older it's easier for them to understand the benefits and why we are reducing their sugar intake. George has quite a bit of anxiety and it has also seemed to improve with less sugar in his diet."

"We've cut back on the cereal bars and flavored yogurt for good. I let the kids get the bars once in a while, but they're more like a treat than a breakfast food or regular item now. I noticed how much sugar affected me, so I keep less of it in the house and I'm craving it far less. It was also nice to get my son involved because at 12, I have less influence over his food choices. So it's nice to see him look at the nutritional values to check the sugar count on items."

"As a post-challenge note, my son is still doing very well. He continues to make better food choices. He is eating a lot of fruit and taking water to school daily. Since completing the challenge, I can't recall when he has had cookies, cake or similar sweets. And when my daughter and I were grocery shopping this past weekend and we were in the beverage aisle, I was looking for Diet Coke. She gave me such a hard time. She asked me, 'Why do you need that, Mom?' I bought sparkling water instead."

Is there progress you would still like to make? Now that your family's on a path to sugar reduction, you might find it easier to incorporate some of the Sugarproof strategies without the formality of the 28-Day-Challenge. But if you like the structure of the challenge, that's great, too. The 28-Day Challenge is here for you whenever you need it. You can shift to new goals or firm up some of your old ones. You can also try the 7-Day Challenge to reset the family's habits, especially after the holidays or vacation. Either way, congratulate yourself on your success. By Sugarproofing your kids, you're giving them better health now—and the ability to make better choices for life.

Weekly Reflection Tool:
4-Week Sugar Reduction Challenge

Name: Age:

Week number (circle one): 1   2   3   4

My goals for this week:

1 _____

2 _____

3 _____

4 _____

Here is a place to take notes about reaching your goals. What recipes, gradual changes, or suggested Sugarproof "hacks" did you try? You can jot down notes daily, or once a week at the end of the week:

_____

In terms of my energy levels this week, I have noticed:
- **Less energy**
- **No change**
- **A little more energy**
- **Lots more energy**

_____

In terms of my mood, I have been:
- **In a worse mood compared to normal**
- **The same as usual**
- **A little better mood**
- **A much better mood**

_____

This week I would give myself the following score for my Sugarproof efforts (1 is lowest and 5 is highest [best]):

1   2   3   4   5

Family Experiment
Find Your Sugarproof Sweet Spot

Our Sugarproof Sweet Spot test is an adaptation of a test that research-ers use to identify sweet taste preference. We've modified it so that everyone in your family can become more aware of their own "sweet spot."

The goal is to see if reducing sugar in the diet will help reset your sweet spot, allowing for the enjoyment of familiar foods and beverag-es at much lower, safer, and healthier levels of sweetness. By perform-ing this experiment as a family before and after our 28-Day Challenge, you can measure how much your sweet taste preference has changed. You and your kids will likely be surprised at how quickly you can get used to enjoying less sweet versions of your favorite foods and drinks. Kids as young as three years can be involved in aspects of this chal-lenge, including the shopping, setup, taste testing, and discussion of the results.

Step 1: Choose the Products You Want to Test
Choose either a sugary beverage (a favorite soda, apple juice, lemon-ade, or sports drink) or plain yogurt with no added sugar or sweeteners.

Step 2: Prepare for the Test
If you're testing a beverage, you will need at least 3.5 cups (28 fluid ounces) plus either plain water, or plain sparkling water as a mixer. We suggest using sparkling water as the mixer for soda to match the carbonation. Prepare six cups or glasses and label them one through six.

If you're using yogurt, buy plain yogurt (3 cups total, or around 26 ounces) and a small bottle of maple syrup. You'll need six small con-tainers, also labeled one through six for the samples.

Then prepare the samples using the charts below.

BEVERAGE TEST

Taste Test Number (Sweetness Level)	Dilution Level	Amount of Sweetened Drink	Amount of Water or Sparkling Water
1 (least sweet)	25%	¼ cup	¾ cup water
2	33%	⅓ cup	⅔ cup
3	50%	½ cup	½ cup
4	66%	⅔ cup	⅓ cup
5	75%	¾ cup	¼ cup
6 (most sweet)	100%	1 cup	none

YOGURT TEST

Taste Test Number (Sweetness Level)	Amount of Yogurt	Amount of Maple Syrup
1 (least sweet)	½ cup	None
2	½ cup	½ tsp
3	½ cup	1 tsp
4	½ cup	1½ tsp
5	½ cup	2 tsp
6 (most sweet)	½ cup	2½ tsp

Make a copy of the rating sheet at the end of the chapter for the family.

Step 3: Pretest

Have each member of the family try a sip or spoonful of each of the options. Move through each of them, starting with the least sweet and finishing with the sweetest, with the goal of identifying which is the least sweet option that they still find enjoyable. Help your younger children identify which they like and fill out the sheet with their preference. After completing the pretest, put your results away in a safe place. You'll refer back to them once you complete the 28-Day Challenge.

Step 4: Compare Your Results

FAMILY PRETEST QUESTIONS:
1. What is the lowest level of sweetness that you liked? This is what we call your pretesting sweet spot.
2. How did the ratings of different members of the family compare?
   a. Who preferred the sweetest options?
   b. Who was happiest with the less sweet options?
   c. Did you notice any patterns? Did the ratings vary by gender or age, with the kids liking more sweet things?
   d. Where is the sweet spot for each family member (lowest level of sweetness that you still found enjoyable)?
3. Did your results surprise you?

Step 5: Posttest

Repeat these same tests after the 28-Day Challenge. Do not look at your results from the pretest so that you won't be biased the second time around. After you complete the posttest, get out your pretest results and compare the two.

FAMILY POSTTEST QUESTIONS:
1. Did anyone's pre- and posttest ratings change? If so, how much?
2. Did anyone start to like some of the less sweet options more?
3. Where is your current sweet spot and has it changed since the pretest?
4. What was this experience like for you? Will it change what you select to eat or drink in the future?

Ideas for other taste tests

You can devise similar tests based on other sugary foods and beverages that you'd like to enjoy but at lower levels of sweetness.

- Oatmeal with varying amounts of honey, brown sugar, or maple syrup

- Hot chocolate prepared with varying amounts of powdered mixture
- Tea or coffee with varying amounts of sugar or sweetener added
- Homemade baked goods made with varying amounts of sugar or sweetener
- Chocolate bars with various amounts of cocoa powder (e.g., 35 percent, 50 percent, 70 percent, 85 percent)

Sugarproof Sweet Spot Rating Sheet
Circle One: Pretest Posttest (after 4-week challenge)

FAMILY MEMBER			BEVERAGE TEST: Circle which is the least sweetened option that you still find enjoyable (1 is least sweet and 6 is most sweet):					
Name	Age	Gender						
			1	2	3	4	5	6
			1	2	3	4	5	6
			1	2	3	4	5	6
			1	2	3	4	5	6
			1	2	3	4	5	6
			1	2	3	4	5	6
			YOGURT TEST: Circle which is the least sweetened option that you still find enjoyable (1 is least sweet and 6 is most sweet):					
			1	2	3	4	5	6
			1	2	3	4	5	6
			1	2	3	4	5	6

| FAMILY MEMBER | | | YOGURT TEST: |
Name	Age	Gender	Circle which is the least sweetened option that you still find enjoyable (1 is least sweet and 6 is most sweet):
			1 2 3 4 5 6
			1 2 3 4 5 6
			1 2 3 4 5 6

To view the scientific references cited
in this chapter, please visit us online at
sugarproofkids.com/bibliography.

CHAPTER TEN

Keep This (Not-So-) Sweet Thing Going: How to Grow the Sugarproof Movement

By now, you may have started your Sugarproof journey. But the dilemma we all face is what to do about the larger food environment kids face every day. Sugar is everywhere, and healthy options are not. Food companies rely on consumers staying uninformed. They also rely on the fact that kids like the taste of sweet products and will demand more. And it's not just the United States that suffers from sugar flooding into its food supply. Sugar is a serious global issue. An economic analysis using data from 2014 estimated that globally, adult obesity cost $2.0 trillion annually, or 2.8 percent of the global gross domestic product. These estimates also indicate that lifestyle diseases such as obesity, heart disease, and dementia are now a greater threat to both the developed *and* the developing world than infectious diseases like HIV. In 2018, the World Health Organization reported that "in just 40 years the number of school-age children and adolescents with obesity has risen more than 10-fold" and asserted that "obesity in adulthood is a major risk factor for the world's leading cases of poor health and early death."

One study concluded that 57 percent of two-year-olds today will be obese by the time they're thirty-five years old. That's more than half of today's toddlers.

Sugar is a societal issue. Many of our colleagues and experts in the field agree that the medical, science, and research communities should join forces to create large-scale change in our food landscape. But what kinds of policies would work best? We'll fill you in on what's been tried so far and which strategies show the most promise.

Make Sugary Drinks More Expensive

A lot of time, money, and effort have been spent on developing policies to tax sugar-sweetened beverages and other sugar-sweetened products in an effort to nudge people to consume less. The tax strategy worked well for tobacco and alcohol reduction programs in the past, although there is still debate in terms of how much tax is needed to make an impact on reducing sugary beverage consumption, with estimates ranging from a 10 percent to a 20 percent increase in cost being needed. In most programs, there is a double benefit because the tax that is raised through these efforts is used to support community health/nutrition education programs.

In the United States, the first and one of the most successful programs was implemented in Berkeley, California, in 2015. Instead of directly taxing consumers or retailers, the companies that contract with beverage makers are levied at the rate of one cent per fluid ounce. They're taxed on sugary sodas as well as energy drinks, juices with added sugar, and the sweet syrups that are pumped into coffee drinks. This tax of one cent per fluid ounce has pushed up the cost of these drinks, and it's having an impressive effect. Compared to similar cities nearby, Berkeley residents have cut sugary beverage consumption in half, down from an average of 1.25 times per day at baseline to 0.7 times per day. However, we do not yet have data on whether these changes in sugary beverage consumption will translate to positive health outcomes.

In an effort to reduce soda consumption, several countries have levied sugar taxes at the federal level. Mexico's population consumes more soda per person than any other country in the world. It also suffers from one of the highest rates of obesity and diabetes. In 2013, it introduced a tax of eight cents per liter on carbonated sugary beverages. Follow-up studies show a 6 percent reduction in annual sales just in the first year. Lower-income households saw the even greater reduction rate of 9 percent. One argument against soda taxes is that they'll disproportionately burden families with lower incomes. But there's another way to look at these results: Perhaps this tax, along with related education, have led this group of consumers to make positive dietary changes that will reduce their risk of future health problems.

By reducing our sugary drink consumption, we could reshape our nation's health. A report by the Milken Institute found that if Americans could reduce their sugary drink consumption by three drinks per month by the year 2030, we could reduce the number of obese Americans by 2.6 million. And the savings in health costs would be huge—a projected $40.7 billion in inflation-adjusted dollars. We would love to see more data on the immediate and long-term effects of soda taxes on consumption and health. And, of course, we'd like soda taxes to include drinks made with LCS.

Passing any soda tax is an uphill battle. Sugar refiners, the corn industry, and soda manufacturers are politically well connected and will fight hard against a tax. In the state of California, the American Beverage Association, a lobbying group for big soda companies, has more than tripled its spending from $200,000 per year in 2015 to just over $700,000 in 2018. It spent almost $300,000 in the first quarter of 2019 alone. Their lobbying was so powerful that in 2018, California passed a new ballot initiative that bans any new local soda taxes in the state until 2031. And companies like Coca-Cola actively try to influence public policy either through lobbying groups like the American Beverage Association or by direct influence of public health policy. For example, Coca-Cola actively engages with organizations like the Centers for Disease Control and Prevention and the World Health Organization to influence policy, trying to shift focus and blame away from sugary beverages as a health concern.

Make Products with Less Sugar

Even the possibility of a soda tax can have a positive influence on the food industry. Soda taxes, or the threat of a tax, have been indirectly effective—because they incentivize companies to make their products with less sugar. A British sugar tax is directed at products with more than the equivalent of 12 grams of sugar in a 12-ounce serving. As a result, some manufacturers in the industry have already reformulated products so the sugar-per-serving amount is under the taxable limit. In the prestigious medical journal *Lancet Public Health*, a group of researchers used statistical modeling to compare strategies for reducing the amount of sugar consumed in beverages. They found that compared to price increases and marketing changes, reformulating drinks would lead to the most benefits in reducing diabetes and obesity and improving oral health—and that children under the age of eighteen would benefit the most.

A few companies have started to offer alternatives. For example, Honest Kids apple juice is mixed with water; it contains 9 grams of sugar in each pouch. It's still a lot of sugar, but much less than Minute Maid's 100 percent apple juice, which has more than three times the concentration of sugar.

This strategy comes with an obvious danger. During the low-fat craze of the '80s and '90s, the food industry created a whole new market for low-fat foods. Consumers were already becoming used to skim and 2 percent milk, but with reformulation, every grocery store shelf featured low-fat products, from yogurt to salad dressing. This reformulation shows that the industry can and will respond quickly to consumer demand. But as we now know, many of these products contained increased sugar to offset the loss of fat and flavor. This workaround was not healthy for consumers. Reformulation to reduce sugar could head in the same direction if sugar is simply replaced with another sweetener, even if it is lower in calories. Coca-Cola, for example, has taken this approach with its different low-calorie products. Coca-Cola Life reduced sugar by replacing some with stevia; Coke Zero is made with aspartame and AceK; and Diet Coke is made with Splenda. They're all lower in sugar, but they nevertheless contain LCS. We need targeted efforts to reduce sugars *and* sweetness.

Demand Food Labels That Tell the Truth

Nutrition labels have long been used as a loophole to hide ingredients, sugars, and other undesirable chemical additives. But what would happen if food-labeling policy could force food companies to tell the truth consistently? When done right, labeling laws can be effective, especially when it comes to warning labels. In 2016, Chile began requiring front-of-package warning labels on products with more added sugar, sodium, saturated fat, or calories than limits set by the Chilean Ministry of Health. These warning labels are already starting to change the public's perception of these food products and how often they purchase them. The program also limits advertising to children, a strategy we'll talk about in a moment. Legislators in the United States have proposed adding warning labels to sugary drinks, but it's been a tough battle.

In the United States, there is still some positive news. As we've discussed, new food labels are being introduced in 2020 and 2021, and they'll be required to list not just total sugar content but also added sugar. Mathematical simulations show that these new labels are projected to prevent approximately one million cases of cardiovascular disease and type 2 diabetes over the next twenty years, with a savings of $31 billion in healthcare costs and $60 billion in total costs to society. The simulations show that these benefits could be doubled if the labels are combined with efforts to reformulate products so that they contain less added sugar. Perhaps one day labels will go a step further to list the different types of sugars, including how much fructose a product contains.

Curbing Advertising

Federal and state governments should support efforts to reduce the marketing of sugary drinks to children and adolescents. In 2009, soda companies spent $395 million directed at marketing to teenagers, and children's exposure to marketing for sodas continues to increase. Food manufacturers have sizable marketing budgets for good reason. They know that when children are exposed to food advertising on TV, they end up consuming more calories. Research has shown that the more kids are exposed to advertisements for sugary products like sodas, the more likely they are to consume them. The United States, however, has been slow to adopt programs to limit food advertising to children, despite recommendations (and even pleas) from many experts, including the American Academy of Pediatrics.

If you think that some of the marketing tactics used for sugary beverages bear close resemblance to the tobacco marketing you recall from your youth, you are not imagining things. The same companies are involved. Iconic logos like the Kool-Aid man and the Hawaiian Punch mascot were created by the same companies that created Joe Camel. Analysis of industry archives has shown, for example, that tobacco executives who were no longer able to strategize how to sell cigarettes to kids instead turned their attention to using the same strategies to hook kids on things like Tang, Capri Sun, and Kool-Aid.

European countries such as Sweden, Norway, and the UK have been more progressive in regulating advertisements to children. The UK, for example, has instituted advertising rules that ban the advertising of foods or drinks that are high in fat, salt, or sugar in any media that targets children younger than sixteen years of age. Moreover, food companies can't use promotions, licensed characters, or celebrities who are popular with children to promote these products—but they *can* use these strategies to help sell foods that are healthier.

Update Our Farming and Food Policies

The United States has used farm policy to ensure a reliable food supply. But agriculture today isn't the same as it was in the 1970s. Seed and equipment technology have made the American farmer more efficient at food production than any other country in the world. It is time to reform US farm policies and/or federal food programs. We need to reduce the incentives to produce foods that harm children's health.

Currently, the government pays farmers a subsidy to grow corn, which in turn encourages the farmers to grow more. Excess corn is used to make corn syrup. This overproduction means that sweeteners such as corn syrup, corn syrup solids, and HFCS are available as a cheap additive for manufacturers to use in food products ranging from infant formula to sodas and fruit drinks and salad dressings. We need to reform food subsidy policies as well as policies that regulate the use of HFCS in food products. Wouldn't it be great if fruits and vegetables were subsidized instead? Better incentives to produce healthy foods would lead to lower prices, giving everyone more options for eating well.

We should also revisit federal food programs that assist low-income families, such as Women, Infants, and Children (WIC) and the Supplemental Nutrition Assistance Program (SNAP). We could improve children's health by promoting items that follow low-sugar guidelines, ensure access to healthy food, and discourage sugary beverages. We've already made a start. For example, WIC (which provides supplemental nutrition to low-income children ages one through five) does not include sodas, although they do still include 100 percent juice in their programs as well as infant formula with added sugars. Standards for subsidized school meals are improving, but fruit juice and flavored milk under some circumstances are still allowed. SNAP, which is also known as the food stamp program, provides food for twenty-three million children—but, unfortunately, it has not yet addressed issues related to food quality, and participants can use these vouchers for sweet items like soda. Believe it or not, SNAP dollars (your tax money) pay for twenty million servings of sugary beverages at a cost of $11 million *per day*. Federal food-assistance programs are relatively easy targets for policy change, and we would like to see this prioritized.

Build a Better Default Menu

In an ideal food environment, sugar would not be so widely available to kids.

Dr. Robert Lustig, a professor of pediatrics at the University of California, San Francisco, describes the similarities between sugar, alcohol, and tobacco in his 2013 book *Fat Chance: Beating the Odds Against Sugar, Processed Food, Obesity, and Disease.* Each substance is widely available, addictive, can be abused as a drug, and has toxic effects when used in excess. Therefore, he proposes, we should treat sugar the way we do alcohol and tobacco, and restrict its access for minors. Of course, it's harder to regulate food, because it's essential for living. A good place to begin, though, is with restaurant menus. Children's menus often feature dessert and sweetened drinks that come free with the meal. Some industry groups are developing new policies that put limits on what's available to kids at restaurants. California recently passed a law called "Healthy by Default Kids' Meals," which went into effect on January 1, 2019. This new law makes water or milk the default drink choice offered with all restaurant kids' combo meals that include a beverage. The law determines what is advertised and offered, but parents retain the ability to request an alternative beverage at no additional charge. This is a simple approach and can be very effective at nudging people toward healthier choices.

What Can You Do Now, as an Individual?

Even if new policies pass, industries can be slow to change. So what can you do to create change? What can you and your kids do to sustain and build a Sugarproof movement? As parents, consumers, and family members, we can take immediate responsibility for improving the American diet through actions such as:

- What we purchase, whether at the grocery store, restaurant, or coffee shop.

- What we eat during pregnancy and what we feed infants and children who are too young to make choices for themselves. We need to disrupt the intergenerational transmission of poor nutrition, obesity, and chronic disease.

- What we teach our children about food, specifically about sugar.

- What habits we model in our own homes and when out with our children.

The good news is that the healthy food movement is catching on, so no one has to walk this path alone. Despite all the complexities and understandings about what constitutes a healthy diet, there is one simple common denominator: Almost everyone agrees that reducing sugar would be a good place to start.

We hope that more and more people will recognize that they and their children will be healthier if they reduce sugar. But even if people understand the problem, they may not know what they could do to make changes. We wrote this book to provide the knowledge, tools, and inspiration for individual and family-based changes when it comes to sugar. Beyond that, we hope to empower families to oppose a food system that pushes sugar on kids at every turn. Here are some ways you can take the Sugarproof movement from your home and into the community:

- Support ballot initiatives for positive food-policy change whether at your school or in your community or state.

- Be vocal within your own communities about foods available in your local schools, churches, stores, and community groups.

- Give non-sugary gifts. Instead of chocolates or candy or cookies, try fun, insulated water bottles, lunch boxes, glass water bottles for the fridge, and other useful kitchen items.

- Subscribe to a local Community Supported Agriculture (CSA) program.

- Support your kids when they advocate for non-sugar treats to their friends, coaches, and teachers in their communities and schools.

- Be creative in the kitchen and share your successes through our online community on our website at www.sugarproofkids.com, or on Facebook, Pinterest, Instagram, or Twitter.

- Plant fruit trees at home and in the community or schoolyard. Next time your school asks for a monetary donation, offer to plant fruit trees instead or help fund a school garden. As an added benefit, trees and gardens help fight climate change.

- Host a savory bake sale, or bring Sugarproof treats to the next school or community fund-raiser.

- Challenge other families to see who can complete the no-added-sugar challenge.

- Encourage your local coffee shops and restaurants to modify or add menu item options that are low in added sugar.

Sweet treats bring joy and pleasure. They're an important part of celebration, community, and childhood. Sugarproof isn't about quitting sugar entirely. It's about becoming less reliant on sweet foods and drinks as daily staples. As you find yourself moving away from sugar, you'll tip your family's balance away from processed foods and toward more whole foods. When things start to feel out of balance in your family, you will know to take a step back, reflect, and reboot using some of the strategies we suggest in this book.

Reducing sugar in your family's diet is a long-term strategy that will yield direct results when it comes to health. The best news is that you can start right now to improve your home food environment and raise your kids to be Sugarproof. Reducing sugar consumption will go a long way in shaping the overall health of the next generation. And ultimately it will make us a society where good food and good health are the norm. You're ready to raise your kids with the tools to make healthy eating choices on their own, to become their own advocates, and to shape the environment in which they will eventually raise their own children.

To view the scientific references cited
in this chapter, please visit us online at
sugarproofkids.com/bibliography.

Part Three

The Sugarproof Kitchen: Recipes and Tips

We are excited to share this collection of recipes with you. It's a combination of some of our family favorites and new recipes that Emily developed for this book. Our basic food philosophy is to keep things simple and based on whole foods. We aim to provide you with easy recipes, tips, and hacks that reinvent classic family food and expand family repertoires for flavorful, healthy eating without added sugars.

We follow these nutritional principles for our recipes:

1. Avoid added sugars and low-calorie sweeteners.
2. Reduce simple carbohydrates that rapidly break down into sugar.
3. Increase protein and dietary fiber to help regulate blood sugar and energy levels and to keep hungry kids feeling satisfied for longer.

Many of the recipes are savory and do not require anything sweet in them, though interestingly if you were to buy these types of foods premade from the grocery store or order them at a restaurant, you would likely find some type of added sugar or sweetener in them. Examples include soups, pasta sauce, and sausages. That's why we have developed our own versions, which you can rely on for easy, nutritious meals at home. For our sweet recipes, such as the muffins, cakes, and granola, we sweeten only with whole fruits (either fresh or dried). This retains the fiber of the fruit and helps lower the glycemic index of the final product. We also use whole grains to increase fiber and we further lower their glycemic index by adding in protein and healthy sources of fat. We are not saying that you can't ever use some added sugar or refined flours when you cook or bake, but we hope to make the point that it's not always necessary.

In addition to thinking about the nutritional quality of the recipes, we kept several practical considerations in mind to make sure we cater to busy families and individual needs:

1. **SIMPLICITY:** recipes that can be made quickly or in advance to create a foundation for healthy meals throughout the day and week.

2. **VERSATILITY:** recipes that work across all meals, including breakfast, lunch, snacks, and dinner, which allows for prepared foods to be used interchangeably.

3. **FLEXIBILITY:** recipes with ideas for variations and substitutions to meet individual needs and food preferences in your family.

We are busy parents ourselves, and we know it's a constant juggle to feed a family well. While we do make a conscious choice to invest time in cooking, we also look for ways to save time—this was central to the thought process for developing these recipes. For example, for muffins, we use a method where you put all of the ingredients into the blender rather than using two mixing bowls for dry and wet ingredients. The fewer steps the better, and the fewer dishes to wash. We also hope to save you time by giving you recipes that can be used interchangeably between meals. For example, you can make the Fuss-Free Frittata (page 279) for dinner, and any leftovers can be eaten cold the next day for breakfast or sent to school as part of a packed lunch. You can use many of the recipes as a basis for multiple meals. For example, if you make the Basic Sugarproof Pasta and Pizza Sauce (page 336), you can also use it to make a simple shakshuka dish by warming it and poaching eggs in it. Or you can prep things like our Roasted Vegetable Master Recipe (page 312) and our Super Green Sauce (page 338) early in the week and then use them to assemble a quick grain bowl dinner by adding your favorite cooked grain and protein of choice. While you may not have time for projects in the kitchen every week, you might have time to make some of our recipes in bulk and freeze them. Finally, we know that it can be complicated to cater to various preferences and food restrictions of family members. Because we understand these situations, we tried to make our recipes as flexible as possible so that you can adapt them to what your family likes and can eat.

Ideas for Involving Your Kids in Trying These Recipes

Kids will be even more receptive to trying these foods if they help prepare them. Here are some ideas for tasks kids can help with in the kitchen. If you set them up with a little station and an age-appropriate task, you can actually put them to work, which helps familiarize them with the ingredients, keeps them occupied, and can even save you time when cooking. Even my (Emily's) five-year-old is a helpful prep cook. He snaps the tough parts off of asparagus spears, peels carrots and cucumbers, and picks leaves off the stems from herbs like parsley or cilantro. The first few times he did each of those tasks, he needed my help, but now all I have to do is set him up, and he works independently.

Kitchen Tasks for Kids
Fruit and Vegetable Prep:
- Wash produce.
- Pick cherry tomatoes or grapes off the stems.
- Cut softer fruits or vegetables like cucumbers, peppers, mushrooms, melons, pineapple, persimmons, or pears. Some pre-prep may be required on your part.
- Prepare lettuce: wash and dry lettuce using a salad spinner and tear it into pieces.
- Snap the ends off of green beans or asparagus.
- Snap florets off stalks for broccoli or cauliflower (cut the stalk off near the florets to give them a head start).

- Shell beans or peas.
- Peel the outer leaves off Brussels sprouts.
- Strip kale off the ribs.
- Baste vegetables with oil using a brush to prep for roasting.
- Husk corn.
- Arrange cut, raw fruit or vegetables on a plate for serving.

Prep for Seasonings and Other Ingredients for Sides or Main Dishes:

- Peel garlic.
- Smash garlic, ginger, or spices with a mortar and pestle.
- Chop onion, nuts, or other ingredients using a pull chopper tool.
- Weigh or measure dry goods like rice, lentils, or pasta.
- Pick leaves off the stems for fresh herbs: rosemary, basil, thyme, basil, cilantro, parsley, etc.
- Sprinkle herbs or spices over dishes.
- Mix and roll dough for fresh pizza or pasta.
- Whisk vinaigrette.
- Spoon dips or dressings into ramekins.

Baking Prep:

- Crack and beat eggs (may need extra supervision depending on age).
- Measure or weigh ingredients.
- Mix or whisk batter.
- Add ingredients to the blender and blend for quick cakes and muffins.
- Spoon batter into muffin cups.
- Roll dough with a rolling pin.

Safety note: Before allowing your kids to use knives, teach them basic knife safety like making sure that what they are cutting sits flat on the cutting board and does not wobble and tucking in fingertips on the opposite hand they are using to hold the knife. Find an age-appropriate knife for your child, but whatever you pick, make sure that it actually cuts through what you are having them cut. Dull knives can actually be more dangerous than sharp ones, and frustrating as well. Very young kids can cut soft things like melon with table knives. Older kids can use full-sized sharp knives to cut hard things if taught to hold them properly, and can also use other tools, like a mezzaluna, for chopping.

Kitchen Tools

These are the tools we use most in our kitchens. Often there is a workaround if you don't have all of these items, but you may want to consider investing in some of them if you plan to increase the amount of cooking you do as a family.

- Sturdy cutting boards
- Paring knife
- Chef's knife
- Pull chopper tool
- Vegetable peeler
- Pizza cutter
- Garlic press
- Strainer/colander
- Salad spinner
- Microplane grater and/or citrus zesting tool
- Grater (box or flat)
- Wok
- Heavy bottomed stockpot or Dutch oven
- Medium frying pan (preferably stainless steel)
- Large cast-iron skillet
- Measuring cups
- Measuring spoons
- Whisk
- Medium/large mixing bowl
- Rolling pin
- Food processor
- High-speed blender
- Sheet pan
- 9-inch springform cake pan
- Baking pans (one 9-inch round or square and one 9x13-inch)
- Muffin tins (regular or silicone)
- Rubber scraper
- Spatula
- Glass storage containers with lids
- Small jars with lids for chia puddings and yogurt cups
- Silicone Popsicle molds and wooden Popsicle sticks

Sugarproof Pantry List

Here is a list of some of the items we regularly stock in our pantries, which form the basis for many of our recipes.

SEASONINGS:

- Olive oil
- Coconut oil
- Sesame oil
- Balsamic vinegar
- Apple cider vinegar
- Tamari
- Furikake
- Maldon salt or other high-quality sea salt
- Assorted spices (e.g., cinnamon, ginger, nutmeg, turmeric, oregano, smoked paprika, ancho chili powder, cumin, black pepper, garam masala, fennel seeds, sage, etc.)

OTHER PANTRY ITEMS IN CANS/CARTONS/JARS:

- Tomato passata (Italian sieved tomatoes)
- Diced canned tomatoes
- Tuna packed in olive oil
- Capers
- Chickpeas
- Other canned or dried beans (black, kidney, etc.)
- Dry lentils
- Coconut milk

DRIED FRUITS/NUTS:

- Dried unsweetened fruit (e.g., dates, dried plums, golden raisins, figs, cherries)
- Raw nuts (e.g., almonds, pecans, hazelnuts, pistachios, walnuts)
- Raw seeds (sesame, flax, pumpkin, chia, hemp, poppy)
- Tahini
- Nut butters (almond, cashew, peanut, etc.)

FLOURS:

- Almond flour
- Buckwheat flour
- Spelt flour
- Coconut flour
- Whole-wheat flour

BAKING STAPLES:

- Baking soda
- Baking powder
- Unsweetened cacao/cocoa powder
- Vanilla extract (no added sugar)

GRAINS/GRAIN PRODUCTS:

- Farro
- Brown rice
- Black rice
- Quinoa
- Rolled oats
- Steel-cut oats
- Whole-grain pasta
- Cornmeal

OTHER:

- Dried wakame (seaweed)

BEVERAGES:

- Herbal teas
- Sparkling water

Sugarproof Recipe Index

Fuss-Free Frittata

SERVES 4

Frittata is great for a high-protein, vegetable-packed breakfast. It's flexible and allows you to use the vegetables you have on hand, even those leftover from dinner. This method is especially easy and "fuss-free" in that it does not require flipping and it uses only the oven. You can do other things while it bakes without having to attend to it. It's also easy to make this frittata the day before and warm it before serving or enjoy it cold at breakfast or lunch.

2 tablespoons butter (can substitute olive oil or use half of each)

4 large eggs, beaten

1 cup cooked, chopped, and drained vegetables of choice like broccoli, peppers, mushrooms, spinach, or zucchini

⅓ cup grated Parmesan or other cheese of choice (optional)

Generous pinch salt

Fresh herbs like chives, basil, or parsley (optional)

1. Preheat the oven to 350°F.

2. Put the butter/olive oil in a 9-inch round glass pie/Pyrex pan and place it in the oven until the butter is melted and is just starting to sizzle, 2 to 3 minutes. The pan needs to be hot so the eggs don't stick in the next step.

3. Remove the pie pan from the oven, tilt the pan around to distribute the butter/oil, and gently pour in the eggs.

4. Sprinkle the chopped vegetables over the eggs, followed by the cheese (if using), and a pinch of salt.

5. Return to the oven and bake for about 10 minutes or until the frittata puffs up slightly and is golden brown and set.

6. Remove from the oven and sprinkle with fresh herbs (if using). Let the frittata cool slightly before attempting to cut it or remove it from the pan.

NUTRITION FACTS PER SERVING: Calories 170 Total Fat 13g Protein 11g Total Carbohydrate 3g Dietary Fiber 1g Total Sugars 1g Added Sugars 0g

*NOTE: recipe analyzed using broccoli and Parmesan cheese.

Popeye Scramble
with Sweet Potato Toast

SERVES 4 (SMALL PORTION)

Many kids like scrambled eggs, and adding spinach to them is a way to make them even more nutritious. You can keep this recipe simple, or you can add extra toppings like cheese, avocado, or chopped cherry tomatoes. One of the ways we like to serve this is with sweet potato toast, which adds even more nutrition to the meal (recipe follows).

2 tablespoons butter (or oil of choice)

3 cups fresh baby spinach, washed and dried

4 large eggs

Salt

Freshly ground black pepper (optional)

1. Heat the butter or oil over medium heat in a frying pan.

2. Add the spinach and cook, stirring occasionally, until wilted.

3. Meanwhile, beat the eggs.

4. Raise the heat slightly and add the eggs to the pan. Once they have begun to cook, move them around with a spatula to scramble them. Continue until they are cooked through.

5. Season with salt. Add pepper if desired.

NUTRITION FACTS PER SERVING: Calories 130 **Total Fat** 10g **Protein** 7g **Total Carbohydrate** 2g **Dietary Fiber** 1g **Total Sugars** 0g **Added Sugars** 0g

Sweet Potato Toast

SERVES 4 WITH 2 SMALL SLICES EACH

Peel a medium sweet potato and slice it into thin, even slices (approximately ¼ inch thick). Toast them in your toaster until they are browned (this can take up a few cycles of toasting). Trim/break off any burnt edges. Spread with butter or brush with olive oil, sprinkle lightly with salt, and serve.

NUTRITION FACTS PER SERVING: Calories 45 **Total Fat** 2g **Protein** 1g **Total Carbohydrate** 7g **Dietary Fiber** 1g **Total Sugars** 1g **Added Sugars** 0g

Egg in a Basket

SERVES 1

This recipe is fun and easy, and a great way to get kids excited about eating an egg at breakfast. Kids especially love to help cut out the circle in the toast. Depending on the size of your frying pan, you may be able to do two slices of bread/eggs at once. If you want an even easier concept for an egg in a basket, fry or scramble an egg and put it inside a piece of toasted pita bread.

1 slice of bread, preferably whole-grain

2 teaspoons butter

1 large egg

Salt to taste

1. Place the slice of bread on a cutting board or plate. Using a drinking glass or a round cookie cutter, cut a hole in the center of the bread. (You can cut the hole with a knife if you can't find a suitable glass.) Remove and set the cut circle aside.

2. Melt the butter in a frying pan. Add the slice of bread and allow it to warm for a minute. Alongside, add the round piece of bread you cut out and toast it in the pan as well.

3. Gently crack the egg in the center of the hole. Break the yolk if you prefer it fully cooked.

4. Allow the egg to cook halfway, and then using a spatula, flip the toast over to allow the egg to cook on the other side to desired doneness for the yolk. Flip the circle cut from the bread as well to get it nice and toasty, too. Sprinkle lightly with salt.

5. Serve the egg in the basket with the circle of bread alongside. For those who enjoy runny yolks, the circle is nice for dipping.

NUTRITION FACTS PER SERVING: Calories 270 Total Fat 14g Protein 11g
Total Carbohydrate 24g Dietary Fiber 0g Total Sugars 0g Added Sugars 0g

Homemade Fennel Sausage Patties

SERVES 6 WITH 2 PATTIES PER PERSON

Are you sold on having a high-protein breakfast but getting bored with eggs? Try adding these flavorful homemade sausage patties into the morning rotation. They are healthier than processed breakfast meats, which usually contain sugar and preservatives. You can make these ahead of time, freeze them, and reheat them for a quick addition to breakfast. They also make for a nice dinner, with roasted vegetables or with pasta, like our Broccoli and Sausage Pasta (Pasta Broccoli e Salsiccia) (page 301). The seasonings listed below are all optional, and you can change them according to your own tastes.

1 pound ground meat of choice (turkey, pork, chicken, lamb, or beef)

1 small onion (or two shallots), finely chopped

1 to 2 cloves garlic, finely chopped

1 teaspoon fennel seeds

½ teaspoon sage

½ teaspoon oregano

½ teaspoon salt

¼ teaspoon pepper (black or white)

¼ teaspoon red chili flakes

1 tablespoon olive oil (or other cooking oil)

1. In a large bowl, mix together ground meat, onion, garlic, fennel, sage, oregano, salt, pepper, and chili flakes.

2. Shape the mixture into thin patties (about 2½ inches in diameter and ½ inch thick), making about 12.

3. Heat the oil in a frying pan over low to medium-low heat. Once the oil is hot, add the sausages; if the oil is not hot enough, the sausages will stick. You can do a test by putting a tiny pinch of the meat into the pan and see if it starts to sizzle.

4. Fry the sausages slowly, making sure they are well browned on one side before flipping them over. Depending on your pan, this will take about 7 minutes per side to cook throughout.

5. Transfer them to a serving plate.

6. These can be stored in the refrigerator for up to 3 days and rewarmed in a pan or in the oven. Or they can be cooled and frozen for up to 4 months. We prefer to brown the sausages before freezing them as we find this easier for reheating in a hurry, but you can also freeze them raw.

NUTRITION FACTS PER SERVING: Calories 180 Total Fat 10g Protein 21g
Total Carbohydrate 2g Dietary Fiber 0g Total Sugars 1g Added Sugars 0g

Three, Two, One... Crepes!

MAKES ABOUT 10 CREPES

This recipe has only three ingredients in the proportion of 3, 2, and 1 (plus a pinch of salt). And each crepe takes less than three minutes to cook. You can make the batter the night before and cook the crepes fresh in the morning. Or cook them in advance and simply warm them when you are ready to eat them for a quick breakfast, lunch, or dinner. The possibilities for fillings are endless. We love savory fillings like wilted spinach, avocado, mushrooms, caramelized onions, Emmental, brie, ricotta, fried or scrambled eggs, and smoked salmon. Sweet fillings are also delicious: fresh pear, banana with almond butter, a simple fruit compote (see Simple Fruit Compotes, page 339), or fresh berries with ricotta cheese, cottage cheese, or any thick plain yogurt.

3 large eggs

2 cups milk of choice (cow or plant-based like unsweetened almond milk)

1 cup flour of choice (We prefer buckwheat. This also works with an all-purpose gluten-free flour. You can mix flours as well.)

Generous pinch of salt

Butter or oil of choice for cooking

1. Crack the eggs and put them in the blender. Add the milk, flour, and salt. Blend until smooth. If time allows, allow the batter to rest for at least 20 minutes or overnight. (This is especially helpful if using buckwheat.) Otherwise, just mix and go. Before you begin cooking, whisk or stir the batter to be sure that the flour hasn't settled to the bottom.

2. Heat a shallow frying pan (approximately 8 inches wide) over medium heat. We use a stainless steel pan, but many people prefer a nonstick pan, as it can be easier to work with. For extra-efficient crepe preparation, get two pans going at once. Be sure the pan is nice and hot, which helps prevent sticking.

3. Put a small pat of butter or oil of choice in the pan, and swirl it around.

4. Add about ⅓ cup of batter to the pan and quickly tilt the pan around to make the batter cover the entire bottom surface.

5. Allow the crepe to cook for a few minutes until bubbles form and the edges start to look dry. Loosen the crepe around the edges with a spatula, and then flip it over to cook for 1 minute more on the other side. Don't be discouraged if your first crepe doesn't come out right. They tend to get easier to cook as you go. Continue cooking the rest of the crepes, occasionally whisking or stirring the batter to prevent settling, and adding small amounts of butter or oil to the pan as you go. You can pile the crepes on a plate, as they do not tend to stick to one another.

6. If using vegetable fillings like sautéed mushrooms or spinach, you can add these to the crepe while it is in the pan, along with cheese, if desired, to melt it. Fold it over and serve. Or you can bring a stack of plain crepes to the table and serve them with other fillings like avocado and smoked salmon, or berries or sliced fresh fruit with nut butter or cottage cheese.

7. Stack any leftover crepes and store them in your refrigerator or freezer in a ziplock bag or other container and save for future use. You can warm them singly in a frying pan, or warm a stack of them in the oven by placing them in a baking dish and covering them with aluminum foil so they do not dry out while reheating.

VARIATION·
For green crepes, add a handful of fresh spinach or arugula leaves to the blender when making the batter.

NUTRITION FACTS PER SERVING (1 CREPE): Calories 110 **Total Fat** 5g **Protein** 5g
Total Carbohydrate 11g **Dietary Fiber** 2g **Total Sugars** 2g **Added Sugars** 0g

Berry Dutch Baby

SERVES 6

This recipe is an easy way to make a pancake-type breakfast without having to hover over the stove. It is impressive and exciting to bring the puffed-up, jammy pancake to the table for serving. The use of lots of berries adds natural sweetness, making it easier to skip the maple syrup. The batter can be made the night before (mixing all ingredients together except the butter and storing in the fridge).

3 large eggs

½ cup milk

½ teaspoon vanilla extract

½ cup all-purpose flour, preferably whole-grain (gluten-free all-purpose flour also works here)

½ teaspoon salt

3 tablespoons unsalted butter

1 cup berries of your choice (blueberries and/or blackberries work very well)

1. Preheat the oven to 425°F.

2. In a medium mixing bowl, beat the eggs and whisk in the milk and vanilla. Add the flour and salt and whisk again.

3. Put the butter in a large cast-iron pan and warm it in the oven for 3 to 5 minutes, until melted.

4. When the butter is melted, swirl around the butter to make sure the pan is fully coated and then pour the butter into the batter and whisk to combine.

5. Pour the batter/butter mixture back into the pan and top with the berries.

6. Put the pan back into the oven to bake for 15 minutes. The "crust" should be nice and brown, the base puffed up, and the fruit bubbly and jammy on top.

7. Slice and enjoy.

VARIATIONS:

This can also be made with other types of fruit such as bananas or peaches, or it can be made into a savory breakfast by adding toppings such as roasted vegetables, smoked salmon, or ham.

NUTRITION FACTS PER SERVING: Calories 150 Total Fat 8g Protein 5g
Total Carbohydrate 12g Dietary Fiber 1g Total Sugars 3g Added Sugars 0g

Blueberry Banana Muffins

MAKES 12 MUFFINS

A blueberry muffin from a coffee shop can easily have up to 30 grams of added sugar whereas one of these Sugarproof muffins only has 7 grams of sugar, all from the banana and the blueberries. Because the batter is made with oats and almond flour, they are high in fiber and also in protein. Making the batter in the food processor (or a blender) is the secret to giving them a light texture. But if you don't have one, you can still make these by mashing the banana by hand and buying pre-ground oat flour (or using whole rolled oats) and mixing the batter in a bowl. Note that this recipe was tested with medium to large bananas. If using very small ones, consider adding an extra half or whole banana.

Oil of choice for greasing the muffin tin

¾ cup rolled oats (not instant)

½ teaspoon salt

½ teaspoon baking soda

4 large eggs

4 medium to large ripe bananas

Zest from 1 lemon (optional)

1 teaspoon vanilla extract, preferably with no added sugar

2 cups almond flour

1 cup fresh blueberries, rinsed and well-drained (you can substitute frozen)

1. Preheat the oven to 350°F.

2. Grease a 12-muffin pan with an oil of choice, or use paper liners.

3. Put the oats, salt, and baking soda in the bowl of a food processor or blender. Process them into an even-textured flour.

4. Add in the eggs, bananas, lemon zest if using, and vanilla and process until smooth.

5. Add the almond flour and process until well-combined.

6. Pour or spoon some batter into each muffin cup, filling them halfway. Sprinkle a few blueberries in each cup, then distribute the rest of the batter. Top the muffins with the remaining blueberries, gently pressing them into the batter to anchor them.

7. Bake for about 30 minutes, or until golden brown and a toothpick inserted into the middle comes out clean.

8. Allow to cool for about 10 minutes before removing from the pan.

VARIATIONS:

Gluten-free muffins: Use gluten-free rolled oats.

Nut-free muffins: Substitute the almond flour for ½ cup coconut flour. (You need much less coconut flour, as it absorbs moisture.)

Grain-free muffins: Omit the oats and increase the almond flour to 2½ cups.

Other berry muffins: Replace the blueberries with other berries of choice, such as strawberries or raspberries.

Banana-nut muffins: Omit the blueberries and add ½ cup chopped nuts like walnuts or pecans in their place along with ¼ teaspoon of a warm spice like cardamom or nutmeg.

Vegan muffins: Replace the 4 eggs with 4 "flax eggs" (make these by mixing 4 tablespoons flax meal with ½ cup plus 2 tablespoons water; let sit for 5 minutes before adding to the batter).

NUTRITION FACTS PER SERVING (1 MUFFIN): Calories 190 Total Fat 11g Protein 7g
Total Carbohydrate 18g Dietary Fiber 4g Total Sugars 7g Added Sugars 0g

Apple Plum Muffins

MAKES 12 MUFFINS

These easy muffins have been a big hit with families who have taste-tested them. You can customize them by leaving the texture of the apples and dried plums coarse, or blending them smooth, which many toddlers and young kids prefer. Adding the extra spices makes these muffins a perfect treat for the fall and holiday season. With 8 grams of total sugar per serving and no added sugar, these muffins are less sweet than typical baked goods, and they are also balanced with 4 grams of fiber and 6 grams of protein.

Oil of choice for greasing the muffin tin

½ cup rolled oats (not instant)

½ teaspoon salt

½ teaspoon baking soda

1 teaspoon cinnamon

¼ teaspoon ground cloves or nutmeg (optional)

2 medium apples (or 3 small), around 12 oz. of whole or 10 oz. of sliced apple

1¼ cups pitted dried plums (prunes)

4 large eggs

1¾ cups almond flour

1. Preheat the oven to 350°F.

2. Grease a 12-muffin pan with an oil of choice or use paper liners.

3. Put the oats, salt, baking soda, cinnamon, and cloves, if using, in the bowl of a food processor or a blender. Process them into an even-textured flour.

4. Core the apples and cut them into slices, but leave the skin on.

5. Add the apples and dried plums to the food processor (or blender) and pulse to chop them into an even texture. Or you can blend them more if you prefer a smooth texture.

6. Add in the eggs and pulse until combined.

7. Add the almond flour and pulse a few more times.

8. Spoon the batter into the muffin pan.

9. Bake for about 30 minutes, or until golden brown and a toothpick inserted into the middle comes out clean.

10. Allow to cool for about 10 minutes before removing from the pan.

VARIATIONS:

Apple Fig Muffins: Replace the dried plums with 1¼ cups dried figs (about 10 large, or 6 oz.).

Gluten-free muffins: Use gluten-free rolled oats.

Nut-free muffins: Replace the almond flour with ⅓ cup coconut flour (you need much less coconut flour).

Vegan muffins: Replace the 4 eggs with 4 "flax eggs" (make these by mixing 4 tablespoons flax meal with ½ cup plus 2 tablespoons water; let sit for 5 minutes before adding to the batter).

NUTRITION FACTS PER SERVING (1 MUFFIN): Calories 100 Total Fat 9g Protein 6g Total Carbohydrate 19g Dietary Fiber 4g Total Sugars 8g Added Sugars 0g

Overnight Steel-Cut Oats, Two Ways

SERVES 1

Steel-cut oats are the healthiest type of oats because they are the least processed and less likely to spike your blood sugar than would rolled oats or instant oats. They do require a longer cooking time than rolled oats, but it is easy to get around this by letting them soak overnight. You can either soak them and heat them up in the morning to serve them warm, or you can eat them cold, which makes for an easy, portable breakfast.

Warm Version

⅓ cup steel-cut oats per serving

⅔ cup (or up to 1 cup) water or milk of choice per serving

1. Put ⅓ cup oats per person in a saucepan.

2. Add ⅔ cup water per person, i.e., a 2 to 1 ratio of oats to water. (Note that if you prefer softer oats, you can increase the liquid to a 3 to 1 ratio, but this will also slightly increase the cooking time the next day).

3. To accelerate the soaking process, you can bring the oats to a boil, remove them from the heat, cover them, and allow them to sit overnight.

4. Otherwise, just add the liquid and let them soak overnight. If using water or plant-based milk, this can stay on the stovetop overnight. If using cow's milk, put the pot in the refrigerator.

5. In the morning, simply put the pot on the stove and heat through to serve. (If you used a 3 to 1 ratio of liquid to oats, you will need to simmer them for a few minutes.)

6. The oats can be naturally sweetened by adding one chopped date per person (or a sprinkle of raisins) before heating, smashing the dates with a fork for even sweetness. Or you can simply top the oats with fresh fruit such as blueberries or banana, a simple fruit compote (see Simple Fruit Compotes, page 339), or other toppings like nuts, cinnamon, or cream.

Cold Version

⅓ cup steel-cut oats per serving

½ to ⅔ cup water or milk of
choice per serving

Optional flavors and sweeteners:
cinnamon, grated apple, raisins,
chopped dates or other dried fruit,
berries, nut butter, or nuts/seeds of
choice

1. Using jars or other portable containers, put ⅓ cup of steel-cut oats in each, followed by ½ to ⅔ cup water or milk of choice. (Choose the amount of liquid based on how milky you like your oats.)

2. Stir in flavorings of choice, close the jars, and store them in the refrigerator overnight (or up to 3 days). These make an easy grab-and-go breakfast. Alternatively, you can make one big container and serve it into bowls the morning of for eating at home.

Note: The texture of the oats will remain fairly firm, which may take a bit of getting used to. If you prefer softer oats, you can substitute Scottish oats (steel-cut oats ground down to a finer grain) or use regular rolled oats.

NUTRITION FACTS PER SERVING: Calories 220 Total Fat 2.5g Protein 7g
Total Carbohydrate 42g Dietary Fiber 6g Total Sugars 1g Added Sugars 0g

*NOTE: recipe analyzed using ⅓ cup oats prepared with water.

Overnight Chia Pudding Cups

SERVES 1

This is an easy make-ahead breakfast that you can prepare directly in individual containers, which can be quickly served or taken with you in the morning. The ingredients listed below are for one serving, so you can measure these quantities into each container/jar, making as many servings as you want. The base recipe can be made in advance and stored in the fridge for a few days, and you can add fresh toppings the day of, if desired.

¾ cup unsweetened milk of choice

1 tablespoon chopped dates or raisins

¼ teaspoon vanilla extract (optional)

2 to 3 tablespoons chia seeds, depending on desired consistency for the pudding

Optional toppings to be added the next day:

Berries or chopped fresh fruit

Chopped nuts of choice

Sugarproof granola (see Sugarproof Granola and Granola Thins, page 295)

1. Add the milk, dates, vanilla if using, and chia seeds to a mug, bowl, or jar, putting the chia seeds in last.

2. Stir well.

3. Put in the refrigerator to set overnight.

4. Add any extra toppings of choice and enjoy.

NUTRITION FACTS PER SERVING: Calories 200 Total Fat 12g Protein 7g Total Carbohydrate 21g Dietary Fiber 13g Total Sugars 7g Added Sugars 0g

*NOTE: recipe analyzed with unsweetened almond milk, 2 tablespoons chia seeds, and 1 tablespoon raisins.

Sugarproof Granola and Granola Thins

**MAKES 4 CUPS OF GRANOLA (16 SERVINGS) OR
AROUND 24 RECTANGULAR GRANOLA THINS**

Granola is a great topping for natural yogurt for a healthy breakfast or snack. Regular commercial granolas have lots of sugar in them, whereas this Sugarproof granola uses dried figs (or other dried fruits) as the sweetener, which also adds extra fiber and other nutrients. This same recipe also makes granola bars, which we like to roll thin, almost like crackers. They are a great snack on their own or dipped in plain yogurt. You can even put them in the toaster and warm them up like you would a toaster pastry and spread with butter, cream cheese, or a nut/seed butter of choice.

1¼ cups dried figs (10 to 12 large, or 6 oz.), or 1¼ cups dried apricots, dried unsweetened mango, or raisins

¼ cup oil of choice, such as coconut or sunflower

1 teaspoon vanilla extract, preferably with no sugar

2 tablespoons flaxseeds (or sesame or hemp)

¼ cup sunflower seeds (or pumpkin)

¼ cup dried, unsweetened flaked coconut

¼ teaspoon salt

¼ teaspoon nutmeg or cinnamon (optional)

2 cups rolled oats (not instant)

Parchment paper (if making granola thins)

METHOD (FOR GRANOLA):

1. Put the figs (or other dried fruit) in a bowl and cover with hot water. Allow to soak for about 20 minutes, until they are softened.

2. Preheat the oven to 300°F.

3. Drain the figs well, remove any tough parts of their stems, and put them in the bowl of a food processor and process them into a paste.

4. Add the oil, vanilla, flaxseeds, sunflower seeds, coconut, salt, and nutmeg if using, and pulse them together to combine.

5. Add the oats and pulse until they are integrated with the other ingredients.

recipe continues

6. Spread the mixture on a rimmed baking sheet and put it in the oven.

7. Bake for 45 to 60 minutes, checking and gently stirring every 15 minutes. The granola is done when it looks golden brown and the clusters feel fairly firm to the touch. They will harden a bit more as they cool.

8. Allow the granola to cool on the pan, and then transfer it to an airtight container for storage, where it will keep for a few weeks.

METHOD (FOR GRANOLA BARS/THINS):

1. Follow steps 1 to 4 above.

2. For step 5, process the oats with the other ingredients for longer, blending continuously instead of pulsing, until the mixture turns into a dough-like consistency. It should feel very slightly damp. If it is dry, add 1 tablespoon water and blend it again until it comes together as a dough, adding an extra tablespoon water at a time if it still seems dry.

3. Remove the dough from the food processor and divide it into two balls of equal size. (To make thicker bars, make just one ball of dough.) Put a piece of parchment paper about the size of a baking sheet on a kitchen work surface. Put one of the balls in the middle of it, cover it with another piece of parchment paper, and flatten it into a disk with your palm.

4. Using a rolling pin, roll the dough over the top of the parchment paper until it is very thin and about the size of a baking sheet. Remove the top layer of parchment paper and transfer the bottom piece of paper with the dough on it onto a baking sheet.

5. Bake for 15 to 20 minutes or until the thins are golden brown. (If making thicker bars, you will need to bake them for around 25 minutes.)

6. Transfer the paper with the baked granola dough to a cutting board and immediately cut it into squares or rectangles using a pizza cutter or a sharp knife. The scraps left around the edges are very tasty, too.

7. If making the thin version, repeat this process with the other half of the dough.

8. Allow to cool and transfer to an airtight container for storage.

9. Thicker bars can be rewarmed in the toaster.

Note: The ingredients are fairly flexible, so if you want to make substitutions like we noted, feel free; just try to keep the same type of ratios of types of ingredients, especially if making the granola thins where the consistency of the dough is important. For example, you could substitute pumpkin seeds for sunflower seeds, or sesame seeds for the flaxseeds, or cinnamon for the nutmeg. To make this recipe gluten-free, simply use gluten-free oats.

NUTRITION FACTS PER SERVING: Calories 130 Total Fat 7g Protein 2g
Total Carbohydrate 17g Dietary Fiber 3g Total Sugars 6g Added Sugars 0g

Acai, Blueberry, and Lemon Smoothie Bowl

SERVES 4 AS A SMALL BOWL

Acai is a fruit that is low in sugar and full of antioxidants. Blueberries also have many beneficial properties, including reducing risk for diabetes. The optional maca powder adds extra fiber, vitamins, and minerals. Serving this smoothie in a bowl with a spoon allows you to appreciate its beautiful colors and also the colorful toppings. To make it a more complete breakfast, add protein-rich toppings like nuts or plain yogurt, or blend a scoop of unsweetened protein powder into the smoothie.

One 3½-ounce package frozen, unsweetened acai (you can substitute this with an additional cup of berries if desired)

2 cups frozen or fresh blueberries (or other berries of choice)

1 frozen banana

1 tablespoon maca powder (optional)

1 cup unsweetened almond milk (or any unsweetened nut milk)

Zest of 1 lemon

Optional toppings/additions:
Toppings are infinite and include other sliced fruit, berries, bee pollen, chopped nuts, seeds like chia or sunflower, dried coconut, or a dollop of plain yogurt.

1. Put all of the main ingredients (not the toppings) in a blender and blend until smooth. The end result should be very thick. Depending on the power of your blender, you may need to pause to scrape down the sides of the jug and blend again. If the ingredients are not mixing, add a splash more of almond milk and try again.

2. Divide the smoothie into bowls, add toppings, and enjoy with a spoon.

NUTRITION FACTS PER SERVING: Calories 100 Total Fat 2.5g Protein 2g
Total Carbohydrate 20g Dietary Fiber 3g Total Sugars 12g Added Sugars 0g

One Big Soup

SERVES 6

This soup is a version of Italian minestrone, which literally means "big soup." The recipe is very flexible, so feel free to customize it according to your family's preferences as well as what's in season. This is a great recipe to make a double batch of and reheat throughout the week for quick meals instead of using convenience foods like canned soups, which often contain sugar and preservatives. For extra flavor, top the soup with grated Parmesan cheese and/or a spoonful of our Super Green Sauce (page 338). To make it more of a complete meal, serve it with garlic toast or a cooked grain such as farro. We like to cook the farro in a separate pot of salted water, drain it, and add it to the soup when serving. Quicker-cooking grains like orzo or pasta can be cooked in the same pot with the soup when reheating it.

3 tablespoons olive oil

1 small onion, diced

3 carrots, peeled and diced

2 stalks celery, diced

One 12-oz. can diced or crushed tomatoes (or chopped fresh tomatoes if in season)

4 cups vegetable broth (homemade or store-bought), plus more if needed

1 bay leaf

1 cup diced potato (around 2 small) or 1 cup cubed butternut squash, optional

Sea salt to taste

One 15-oz. can beans of choice, drained, such as kidney or cannellini or ½ cup beans cooked from dried (optional)

2 cups diced seasonal vegetables such as green beans, zucchini, broccoli, or cauliflower

2 cups (packed) leafy veggies such as kale, cabbage, or chard, with tough stems removed and torn or cut into bite-size pieces

A handful chopped, fresh flat-leaf parsley or basil (optional)

1. In a large, heavy-bottom pot, warm the olive oil over medium heat.

2. Add the onions, carrots, and celery and sauté for about 5 minutes, until the onions are translucent.

3. Add the tomatoes, broth, bay leaf, and the potatoes, if using.

4. Bring to a boil and reduce to a simmer for 15 minutes.

5. Add salt to taste.

recipe continues

6. Add the beans and seasonal vegetables and simmer another 10 to 15 minutes.

7. Add the leafy vegetables and simmer 10 minutes more, adding a little more water or broth if needed.

8. Taste the vegetables to make sure they are tender, and simmer for additional time if not.

9. Serve, sprinkling the fresh herbs on top, if using.

NUTRITION FACTS PER SERVING: Calories 190 Total Fat 7g Protein 6g
Total Carbohydrate 26g Dietary Fiber 7g Total Sugars 7g Added Sugars 0g

Broccoli and Sausage Pasta (Pasta Broccoli e Salsiccia)

SERVES 8

A classic combination used often in Italy, sausage and broccoli complement each other fantastically. This recipe provides a complete family meal, including vegetables and protein, in one serving dish. Even kids who are not usually big fans of broccoli tend to like this pasta. You can either buy Italian sausage, ideally one that does not contain added sugars, or you can use our Homemade Fennel Sausage Patties (page 282). Vegetarians or vegans can use a plant-based sausage of choice.

Sea salt to taste

1 extra-large head of broccoli, approximately 1 lb., or two smaller crowns

1 to 3 tablespoons extra-virgin olive oil

2 cloves garlic (optional)

14 oz. of Italian sausage (6 medium) (You can also use our Homemade Fennel Sausage Patties [page 282], or vegetarian sausages of choice of the same weight)

A pinch of pepperoncino (red pepper flakes) (optional)

1 1-lb. box of pasta of choice, preferably whole-grain (Small shapes like orecchiette and fusilli work well.)

Extra olive or butter for finishing (optional)

Grated Parmesan cheese for serving (optional)

1. Bring a medium to large pot of water to boil (at least 2 quarts). This will be used for both the broccoli and the pasta, one after the other. Salt the water with approximately 1 teaspoon per quart.

2. Wash the broccoli and cut the florets away from the tough part of the stalk. Cut larger florets into pieces.

3. Heat a large skillet over medium heat with 1 tablespoon of olive oil. If using garlic, lightly crush it and add to the skillet.

4. If the sausage has casing, remove it and put just the sausage meat in the skillet. Brown it, breaking it up with a spoon or a fork into small pieces as

recipe continues

it cooks. If the sausage is dry, add an additional tablespoon or two of olive oil.

5. While the sausage cooks, put the broccoli into the boiling water and cook for 3 to 5 minutes, until just tender. Remove it from the boiling water with a slotted spoon and add it directly to the skillet. Do not discard the cooking water.

6. Cook the sausage with the broccoli for 1 to 2 minutes to integrate the flavors, adding a sprinkle of pepperoncino if desired. Turn off the heat and remove the garlic.

7. Add the pasta to the cooking water, paying attention to the time you put it in. Stir occasionally. Check the cooking time on the box/bag of pasta. When it is 2 minutes before the suggested time (close to being done), ladle out ½ cup of the cooking water and reserve it in a cup or small bowl. Then drain the pasta and add the pasta to the skillet.

8. Turn the skillet back on and add a splash of the cooking water to the pasta and stir it in, allowing the pasta to finish cooking and integrate with the sausage and broccoli. Taste it, and add more cooking water if needed, stirring until it is done.

9. Add an additional drizzle of olive oil, if desired, or a pat of butter. You can also mix in grated Parmesan cheese.

10. Transfer the pasta to a serving bowl and serve with extra Parmesan cheese if desired.

Note: if your child is not a fan of broccoli, you can smash it with a fork or even blend it in a blender or food processor before adding it to the skillet in Step 5 to create more of a sauce that does not have individual pieces of broccoli. This is also convenient for very little ones who are weaning.

NUTRITION FACTS PER SERVING: Calories 430 Total Fat 19g Protein 17g
Total Carbohydrate 50g Dietary Fiber 7g Total Sugars 3g Added Sugars 0g

Grilled Halloumi Salad

SERVES 4

Halloumi is a Greek cheese that kids may not have tried but often like upon first bite. It is very firm and tastes great grilled or pan-fried, and it can be made ahead and easily sent in packed lunches. Because it is so salty, it goes especially well with salad. It can take some kids a while to get used to eating salad. Emily's sons started to like it once they tried lamb's lettuce (mâche), which is soft and mild. Other kids like crispy hearts of romaine. Experiment to see which lettuce your kids might be willing to try. Another option is to compose a non-lettuce salad with cherry tomatoes, cucumbers, grated carrot, or other veggies your kids already like. This salad can easily become a main dish, especially if you add some of the optional ingredients listed below.

1 8-oz. package of halloumi cheese

8 cups lettuce of choice

2 tablespoons olive oil for drizzling or to taste

2 teaspoons fresh lemon juice or vinegar of choice for drizzling, or to taste

Pinch sea salt

Other possible additions:

Sliced/cubed raw veggies of choice, such as cherry tomato, cucumber, grated carrot or beet, or avocado

Any roasted or steamed leftover vegetables, such as cauliflower or zucchini

Fruit of choice, such as sliced apple or pear, or pomegranate seeds or berries

Nuts or seeds of choice, such as walnuts or sunflower seeds

Other proteins of choice, such as garbanzo beans (our Crispy Chickpea Snacks, on page 316, are great on salad)

Cooked grains of choice, such as quinoa, couscous, or farro

1. Remove the halloumi from the package and drain any water.

2. Cut the halloumi crosswise into slices that are about ¼ inch thick, making about 8 slices.

3. Heat a grill pan or a frying pan over medium-high heat.

recipe continues

4. Place the halloumi slices in the pan and allow to cook for 4 to 5 minutes, until the liquid that comes out of the cheese dries up and starts to brown.

5. Using a spatula, flip the cheese over, taking care to scrape up the browned bits, which are very tasty.

6. Allow the halloumi to brown on the second side. This is usually much quicker, about 1 minute.

7. Remove the halloumi from the pan and allow to cool on a plate for later use, or directly top with your salad if eating right away.

8. Compose your salad with any of the ingredient ideas above and drizzle with olive oil and lemon juice. Sprinkle lightly with sea salt. Remember that the halloumi itself is already very salty.

NUTRITION FACTS PER SERVING: Calories 260 Total Fat 22g Protein 13g
Total Carbohydrate 3g Dietary Fiber 1g Total Sugars 0g Added Sugars 0g

Miso Soup with Tofu

SERVES 4

Many kids like miso soup when they have it at Japanese restaurants, and it's easy to make from scratch at home. The packets that you can buy of miso soup work in a pinch, but they can have sugar and/or MSG in them, or they can be especially high in sodium. Beyond helping you to avoid these unnecessary ingredients, making your own miso soup allows you to use fresh miso paste, which has probiotic properties. When possible, buy miso paste that is sold in the refrigerated section of the store, as it has live cultures. You can use whichever type you would like for the soup, though white has the mildest flavor, which many kids prefer. Buying miso paste with dashi (soup stock) already in it saves time. You can make other versions of the soup by adding vegetables like spinach, enoki mushrooms, or daikon radish, or other proteins instead of tofu, like egg or clams.

2 tablespoons dried wakame seaweed

4 cups water

¾ cup tofu (you can use silken, medium, or firm, depending on your preference), cubed

3 to 4 tablespoons miso paste with dashi (or make your own dashi using kombu and bonito; see Note)

1 green onion, both white and green parts, finely sliced (optional)

1. If you are not using miso paste with dashi in it, follow the steps in the notes below to make dashi of your own using kombu and bonito flakes.

2. Put the dried wakame in a small bowl and cover with water to rehydrate it and remove any sand or dirt.

3. Bring the water (or prepared dashi) to a boil and turn down the heat.

4. Add the tofu and allow it to warm through. Then add the wakame.

5. Turn off the heat. You do not want to boil the miso paste, which you will add in the next step, or it will kill the beneficial bacteria.

6. In a small dish or in a soup ladle, mix the miso paste with a little of the soup broth to dissolve it. Add it to the pot. If the soup has cooled off, you can gently warm it again, but do not bring it to a boil.

7. Ladle the soup into small bowls and top with the sliced green onion.

recipe continues

Note: If your miso paste does not include dashi, which is a type of stock, you can make your own using kombu, which is a type of thick seaweed, and bonito (smoked tuna) flakes. Take one piece of kombu, approximately 4x6 inches, and wipe it clean with a damp paper towel or cloth. Bring 4 cups of water to a boil in a small pot, reduce the heat to low, add the kombu, and cook for 20 minutes, without boiling. Remove the kombu and add 1 cup of bonito flakes. Boil for 1 minute and then strain out the bonito flakes. Use this broth in place of the 4 cups of water in the ingredient list above. For a vegetarian stock, use just the kombu and skip the bonito.

NUTRITION FACTS PER SERVING: Calories 130 Total Fat 2g Protein 14g
Total Carbohydrate 14g Dietary Fiber 8g Total Sugars 3g Added Sugars 0g

Turmeric Veggie Fried Rice

SERVES 4

This dish is an easy one-pan meal that incorporates turmeric, which has broad anti-inflammatory properties. It's also a great way to use any leftover rice and/or any vegetables you have on hand. If you don't have any leftover rice, you can steam some and spread it out to cool before frying. You can also add other protein, like chicken, shrimp, or tofu, which can be cut in small pieces and fried in the same pan before adding in the vegetables. Any leftovers of this dish also work very well warmed for a complete and nutritious breakfast.

1 to 1½ cups raw, crisp-cooked, or frozen vegetables such as shredded raw cabbage or carrot; fresh spinach; par-cooked broccoli, cauliflower, green beans, snap peas, or kale; or frozen peas

1 teaspoon chopped fresh ginger (optional)

1 clove garlic (optional)

1 green onion (optional)

2 tablespoons coconut oil or other oil of choice

2 large eggs

½ teaspoon dried ground turmeric

2 cups cooked cold rice, preferably brown or other whole grain

2 tablespoons soy sauce or tamari

Black pepper, which helps with absorption of the turmeric, making it more bioavailable (optional)

1. Prepare the vegetables as needed: shred some raw carrot or cabbage, or lightly steam some broccoli, cauliflower, kale, or green beans until par-cooked. Small frozen vegetables like peas can be used straight from the freezer.

2. Chop the ginger, garlic, and/or the white part of the green onion, if using.

3. Heat a wok or large frying pan over medium-high heat and add the oil.

4. Add the ginger, garlic, and green onion to the pan and cook for 1 minute, until fragrant.

5. Add the vegetables and fry them for a minute or two.

6. In a small dish, beat the eggs with the turmeric.

recipe continues

7. Pour the eggs into the pan and allow them to begin to set for a minute or so.

8. Add the rice to the pan before the egg is fully cooked so the egg coats the rice.

9. Stir the rice to soften it and break apart any clumps.

10. Add the soy sauce and stir until integrated, the rice is evenly coated, and the egg is cooked.

11. Top with black pepper if using and serve.

NUTRITION FACTS PER SERVING: Calories 230 Total Fat 10g Protein 7g
Total Carbohydrate 29g Dietary Fiber 3g Total Sugars 1g Added Sugars 0g

*NOTE: recipe analyzed with ½ cup peas, ½ cup carrots, and ½ cup cabbage.

Loaded Veggie Chili

SERVES 8

Packed with a variety of vegetables, this vegetarian chili is full of flavor. The eggplant disappears into the chili and gives it a satisfying texture. You can also modify the vegetables based on what your family likes and what's in season. Ancho is a mild chili that adds flavor without much heat. If you can't find ancho chili powder and decide to use generic chili powder, know that it can vary quite a bit in spice level depending on the brand, so start with much less, taste, and add more if desired. This is a great recipe to make in advance and eat throughout the week or freeze and use when busy. For an especially crowd-pleasing meal, pair it with our Mango Cornbread (page 311).

1 small eggplant (around 11 oz.)

1 medium zucchini (around 9 oz.)

⅓ cup olive oil, plus more as needed

1 medium onion

1 red bell pepper

3 cloves garlic

2 to 4 cups vegetable broth

Two 14.5-oz. cans chopped or crushed tomatoes with their juice

3 tablespoons ancho chili powder

1½ teaspoons ground cumin

1 teaspoon oregano

2 teaspoons sea salt or to taste

¼ teaspoon ground cinnamon

½ teaspoon smoked paprika

1 medium sweet potato (around 11 oz.) (optional)

Two 15-oz. cans beans of choice, such as kidney or black beans, drained

Optional toppings:

Chopped cilantro

Sliced avocado

Wedges of lime

Sour cream or plain yogurt

Grated cheese of choice

1. Cut the eggplant and the zucchini into cubes, around ½ inch in size or smaller if desired.

2. In a large, heavy-bottomed pot or a cast-iron Dutch oven, warm the olive oil over medium heat and add the eggplant and zucchini. Sauté them, stirring occasionally, until they become soft and lightly browned.

3. Put the onion and the bell pepper in the bowl of a food processor and chop them finely. (This can also be done by hand.) Add them to the pot with

recipe continues

the eggplant and zucchini and allow to cook, stirring occasionally, until the onions become translucent. If needed, add a drizzle more olive oil to prevent sticking.

4. Mince the garlic (or press it using a garlic press) and add it to the pot, sautéing for a minute or so until fragrant but not allowing it to brown.

5. Add 2 cups of the broth along with the tomatoes and the spices. Stir well.

6. Add the sweet potato, if using, along with the beans.

7. Allow to simmer for about an hour or until the sweet potato is very tender.

8. Check the chili occasionally and add extra broth if it is looking too thick. If using sweet potato, you will probably need at least 3 cups broth total. Without the sweet potato, 2 cups broth may be sufficient.

9. Taste the chili for salt, adding more if needed, and serve along with any desired toppings.

NUTRITION FACTS PER SERVING: Calories 240 Total Fat 11g Protein 8g
Total Carbohydrate 30g Dietary Fiber 10g Total Sugars 8g Added Sugars 0g

Mango Cornbread

SERVES 12

Many cornbread recipes call for added sugar, and most box mixes already contain it. By blending fresh mango into this recipe, you add natural sweetness and moisture to the cornbread as well as extra fiber and vitamins. It's especially good served with our Loaded Veggie Chili (page 309).

Oil of choice for greasing the pan, skillet, or muffin tin (or use muffin liners)

1 medium mango (approximately 1¾ cups cubed fruit; can substitute frozen)*

2 large eggs

1½ cups buttermilk (or 1½ cups milk plus 1 tablespoon lemon juice left to sit for 5 minutes)

2 cups cornmeal (not instant or precooked)

1 teaspoon baking powder

1 teaspoon baking soda

1 teaspoon salt

1. Preheat the oven to 400°F. Grease a 9x13-inch pan or a 12-cup muffin tin.

2. Peel the mango and cut the fruit away from the seed. Put it in the blender along with the eggs and the buttermilk and blend until smooth.

3. Add the dry ingredients to the blender and blend again until smooth.

4. Pour the batter into the muffin cups or greased pan and bake for 15 to 25 minutes until golden brown and a toothpick inserted in the middle of one comes out clean.

* FOR A PEACH VARIATION:
Substitute the mango for 1¾ cups of sliced peach. This is about 2 large or 3 small peaches. We like to leave the skins on to retain the fiber.

Note: You can make this cornbread in a cast-iron skillet. Prepare the batter as directed then add 3 tablespoons of oil of choice to a skillet. Warm in the preheated oven for 5 to 7 minutes. Remove from the oven, swirl around the oil, pour the batter in, and bake for about 25 minutes or until the cornbread is lightly browned and a toothpick inserted in the middle comes out clean.

NUTRITION FACTS PER SERVING: Calories 150 **Total Fat** 2.5g **Protein** 4g
Total Carbohydrate 27g **Dietary Fiber** 1g **Total Sugars** 6g **Added Sugars** 0g

Roasted Vegetable Master Recipe

SERVES 6

Having roasted vegetables on hand opens up so many possibilities. We suggest firing up the oven at least once a week and roasting trays of whatever you have on hand. Then add them to breakfast frittatas or veggie scrambles, serve them as sides in packed lunches, or add them to pasta or quesadillas for easy dinners. You can even offer them to your kids as a snack while they are waiting for dinner to cook. We offer you a basic recipe here as well as some of our favorite combinations.

6 cups sliced or cubed raw vegetables, such as cauliflower, carrots, zucchini, peppers, sweet potatoes, butternut squash, broccoli, eggplant, tomatoes, red onion, or cabbage

¼ cup oil of choice (we prefer olive oil)

Seasonings of choice, such as smoked paprika, oregano, rosemary, sage, basil, cumin, garlic cloves, or cinnamon (optional)

Sea salt to taste

1. Preheat the oven to 375°F.

2. Spread the vegetables out on a rimmed baking sheet, drizzle with the oil, and use your hands to toss and coat them. (Sliced eggplant is even better if brushed with the oil to evenly distribute it.)

3. Sprinkle with any optional seasonings of choice.

4. Roast for 15 to 40 minutes, depending on the vegetable, until the edges start to look brown and slightly crisp. Of the options listed above, broccoli needs the least time, whereas sweet potatoes would likely need the most, depending on how they are sliced.

5. Remove from the oven and sprinkle with sea salt to taste.

SAMPLE FLAVOR COMBINATIONS:

Cauliflower with smoked paprika (tastes great with a squeeze of lemon after roasting)

Zucchini or carrots with red onion, cumin, and cinnamon

Eggplant and tomato with oregano, basil, and garlic

Butternut squash with rosemary and sage

NUTRITION FACTS PER SERVING: Calories 130 **Total Fat** 9g **Protein** 2g **Total Carbohydrate** 12g **Dietary Fiber** 2g **Total Sugars** 3g **Added Sugars** 0g

*NOTE: recipe analyzed for a mixture of cauliflower, sweet potato, and zucchini.

Roasted Red Cabbage Crisps

SERVES 8

Your kids may not typically like cabbage, but don't let that stop you from trying these out. They are beautifully colored and very satisfying, thanks to their crispiness, and of course the olive oil and sea salt. They are great warm, cold, or at room temperature. You can use them as a side dish at dinner, as a component in packed lunches, or even as a snack. They make a beautiful addition to a grain bowl dinner, and thinly sliced, extra-crispy ones are great on top of soups or salads. Note: Thank you to Kami McClure for the inspiration on this recipe.

1 small to medium head of red cabbage (or green, savoy, or other variety)

¼ to ⅓ cup olive oil (or other oil of choice) for drizzling

Sea salt for sprinkling

1. Preheat the oven to 350°F.

2. Wash the cabbage and pat dry.

3. For regular red or green cabbage, remove any damaged outer leaves and quarter it lengthwise. Trim out the inner core with a single diagonal cut. Turn each quarter onto its side so it doesn't roll, and slice it into ribbons. You can make them as fine/thick as you want.

4. For savoy cabbage, peel off the thicker outer leaves, stack them up in stacks of about 4 leaves, and cut alongside either side of the ribs. Discard the ribs (or feed them to some rabbits), and slice the remaining parts into ribbons. Once you get down to the more tender middle section of the cabbage, treat it as you would a red or regular green cabbage, following step 2 above (i.e., cut it into quarters, slice out the core, and slice into ribbons). Thin ribbons are best for savoy cabbage because it can be tougher than other types.

5. Spread the ribbons out onto 2 rimmed baking sheets, large Pyrex dishes, or any other type of roasting pans. You can usually fit about ½ cabbage on each baking sheet. (If you want them to be extra crispy, only use about ¼ cabbage per baking sheet and make a single layer that will brown more evenly.)

6. Drizzle approximately 3 tablespoons of oil over each pan and toss it with the cabbage using your hands or tongs to distribute the oil.

7. Pop them in the oven and roast for 30 to 45 minutes (depending on how crispy you like them), stirring every 15 minutes.

8. Sprinkle with sea salt and enjoy!

NUTRITION FACTS PER SERVING: Calories 90 Total Fat 7g Protein 1g
Total Carbohydrate 8g Dietary Fiber 2g Total Sugars 4g Added Sugars 0g

Crispy Chickpea Snacks

SERVES 8

These roasted chickpeas are an easy, high-fiber snack that is affordable and great for adding to lunch boxes or satisfying hungry kids after school. You can adapt the seasonings to whatever your child likes, or make them with just olive oil and a pinch of salt. We like using garam masala as the seasoning for a curried version. An Italian version with sage, oregano, and rosemary is also very tasty.

2 15-oz. cans of chickpeas (garbanzo beans)

2 tablespoons olive oil, coconut oil, or other oil of choice

½ teaspoon salt

¼ teaspoon cinnamon (optional)

½ teaspoon ground cumin (optional)

¼ teaspoon chili powder (optional)

1. Preheat the oven to 350°F.

2. Drain the cans of chickpeas well, preferably using a small strainer or colander.

3. Spread the chickpeas on a rimmed baking sheet and dry with a clean kitchen towel or paper towels.

4. Drizzle the chickpeas with the olive oil, shaking to evenly coat them (or brush them with a basting brush).

5. Sprinkle the spices and salt over the chickpeas.

6. Roast in the oven for around 30 minutes, shaking occasionally, until brown and crispy.

7. Allow the chickpeas to cool completely before storing. They keep nicely in a paper bag for a day or two, assuming they have been well-roasted. You can also store them in the refrigerator and either eat them cold or recrisp them in the oven, if desired.

Note: We recommend this snack for older children, as it could be a choking hazard for toddlers.

NUTRITION FACTS PER SERVING: Calories 120 Total Fat 5g Protein 5g
Total Carbohydrate 14g Dietary Fiber 4g Total Sugars 3g Added Sugars 0g

"Fruit on the Top" Yogurt Pots

MAKES 4 POTS

Store-bought yogurt with fruit on the bottom is usually full of added sugars. This simple recipe has no added sugar and is easy to customize based on the fruits your child likes. You can play with the ratio of fruit puree to yogurt to help your child get used to the taste of natural yogurt. One of the options we tested was strawberry/banana, because this flavor is so popular in store-bought versions. Homemade tastes so much fresher—no artificial banana flavor here. As an added plus, the strawberry helps the banana from turning brown. Keep these yogurts in your fridge for up to 3 days for a quick addition to breakfast, for use in a packed lunch, or for a snack. As an alternative to using fresh fruit, you can top the yogurt with homemade fruit compote (see Simple Fruit Compotes, page 339).

The amounts listed are just examples, and you can customize the quantities to the size of your jars/containers and your child's preferences.

1 cup fresh fruit such as strawberry, blueberry, mango, pineapple, cherry, peach, apricot, or banana. (If you use banana, consider mixing it with another fruit or a squeeze of lemon or orange to prevent it from turning brown.)

2 cups natural, plain yogurt with no added sugars

1. Puree the fruit in a food processor or blender, pressing down with a spoon if needed to help it blend. Do not add water.

2. Spoon the yogurt into small jars or ramekins, adding about ½ cup to each. Then top the yogurt with about ¼ cup pureed fruit. You can also stir the fruit through the yogurt if your child prefers a more uniform flavor.

NUTRITION FACTS PER SERVING: Calories 90 Total Fat 4g Protein 4g Total Carbohydrate 8g Dietary Fiber 1g Total Sugars 7g Added Sugars 0g

*NOTE: recipe analyzed for strawberry version.

Tamari-Roasted Sunflower Seeds

SERVES 8

Sunflower seeds that you buy pre-roasted are often oily, oversalted, and sometimes even rancid because they sit on the shelf in the store. It's easy to roast your own seeds at home, and they are a high-protein snack that can be included in lunch boxes even when there is a no-nut policy. They also add a nice crunch to salads and can be used in homemade trail mix. This recipe uses tamari for flavor. Tamari is made from fermented soy beans and is similar to soy sauce, though it tends to be less salty and typically does not contain wheat. Because it is a liquid, it adheres nicely to the seeds. You can also try pumpkin seeds for variety.

1½ cups raw, shelled sunflower seeds or pumpkin seeds   **1 tablespoon tamari**

1. Preheat the oven to 350°F.

2. Spread the seeds out on a rimmed baking sheet.

3. Drizzle the tamari over the seeds and use your hands or a spoon to mix them around and distribute the sauce.

4. Roast them in the oven for 15 minutes or until they are golden brown.

5. Cool them completely and store the seeds in an airtight jar or container. Consume them within a few weeks.

NUTRITION FACTS PER SERVING: Calories 150 Total Fat 14g Protein 5g
Total Carbohydrate 5g Dietary Fiber 2g Total Sugars 0g Added Sugars 0g

Easy No-Bake Energy Bites

MAKES 12 ONE-INCH BALLS/BITES

Energy bites are an easy alternative to granola bars, which are often full of added sugars. Kids tend to enjoy these just as much, especially if they have a hand in making them. They don't require baking, and kids as young as preschool age can help with rolling the mixture into balls. This is a flexible recipe; the amount of the basic ingredients stays the same, so you and your kids can use the recipe as a guide, experiment with new combinations, and have fun naming your new flavors as well. We've given you a few ideas as a jumping-off point. The bites work great in lunch boxes and can be made in bulk and stored in the freezer.

½ cup dried, unsweetened fruit of choice

⅔ cup dry, rolled oats (not instant)

½ cup seeds or nuts of choice

Pinch of salt

2 teaspoons coconut oil (or other oil of choice)

Optional flavorings (see chart on opposite page for ideas)

1 to 4 tablespoons water, as needed

⅓ cup topping of choice for rolling (optional; see chart on opposite page)

1 If your dried fruit is especially hard, soak it in warm water for 10 minutes and drain well.

2. Put the oats, seeds, and salt in the bowl of a food processor and process until finely ground.

3. Add the fruit, coconut oil, and optional flavorings and pulse until the mixture comes together. If your mixture is not blending well, add a tablespoon of water at a time until a dough begins to form.

4. Remove the dough from the food processor and roll into 1-inch balls.

5. Roll in the desired topping, if desired.

6. Store the bites in the refrigerator for up to 1 week or freeze for up to 2 months. They can be taken directly out of the freezer in the morning and placed in a lunch box to enjoy later.

recipe continues

Ideas for flavor combinations:

NAME	SEEDS/NUTS	DRIED FRUIT	FLAVORINGS	TOPPING (optional)
Fig Coconut	Sunflower seeds	Figs	½ teaspoon vanilla extract	Dried grated coconut
Black-and-White Brownie	White sesame seeds	Pitted dates	4 teaspoons unsweetened cocoa and 1 teaspoon finely grated orange zest	White sesame seeds or chopped cacao nibs
Apricot Almond	Almonds	Apricots or half apricots, half dates for a sweeter taste	½ teaspoon lemon zest, ½ teaspoon vanilla extract	Finely chopped almonds
Old-Fashioned Oatmeal Cookie	Walnuts or pecans	Raisins	½ teaspoon cinnamon and ½ teaspoon vanilla extract	Finely chopped walnuts or pecans

NUTRITION FACTS PER SERVING: Calories 110 Total Fat 7g Protein 3g
Total Carbohydrate 9g Dietary Fiber 2g Total Sugars 2g Added Sugars 0g

*NOTE: recipe analyzed for Apricot Almond version.

Quick Carrot Cake Macaroons

MAKES 16 COOKIES

These quick, flour-free cookies are high in protein and fiber and provide kids with long-lasting energy. They're also a great way to sneak in carrot for kids who are unsure of it. If you omit the optional walnuts, these can be packed in lunches for kids who attend schools with no-nut policies.

1½ cups finely grated unsweetened, dried coconut

¼ teaspoon salt

½ teaspoon baking soda

½ teaspoon baking powder

½ teaspoon cinnamon

¼ teaspoon allspice

¼ teaspoon nutmeg

3 large eggs

1 banana (or omit and increase the apples to 2)

1 apple, grated with skin

1 small carrot, grated (about ¾ cup)

½ cup raisins

⅓ cup chopped walnuts (optional)

1. Preheat the oven to 350°F.

2. In a small bowl, mix the coconut, salt, baking soda, baking powder, and spices.

3. In a larger bowl, beat the eggs and mash in the banana.

4. Add the dry ingredients to the wet ingredients, stirring until combined.

5. Add the grated apple, carrot, and raisins.

6. Line a large baking sheet with parchment paper.*

7. Using two soup spoons, transfer the batter onto the parchment and shape in slightly raised mounds, approximately 2 inches in diameter.

8. Bake for about 10 minutes, until deep, golden brown. Allow to cool before removing from the parchment.

*Note that these can also be baked in muffin cups if you don't have parchment paper. Store in the refrigerator for up to 1 week.

NUTRITION FACTS PER SERVING (1 COOKIE): Calories 110 Total Fat 7g Protein 2g Total Carbohydrate 10g Dietary Fiber 2g Total Sugars 6g Added Sugars 0g

Flax Thins Crackers

SERVES 8

Kids love crackers, but they can often be a source of empty calories. The dough for these crackers is made out of flax meal, which provides healthy fat as well as fiber. Grinding your own flaxseeds helps preserve the beneficial qualities of the oil they contain. If you use pre-ground flax meal, try to use it soon after opening the bag and store any leftover meal in the refrigerator in an airtight container to prevent it from going rancid. These crackers work well as a satisfying snack on their own but also can be used to dip in hummus, cream cheese, or other spreads. Some kids prefer them plain, but you can add in spices as desired, such as those listed below for an "everything" version.

1 cup ground (milled) golden flaxseeds

¼ teaspoon sea salt, plus additional for sprinkling on top (optional)

Optional spices (see below)*

⅓ cup water

1 tablespoon olive oil

½ teaspoon apple cider vinegar

*For the "Everything" Version, add in:

½ teaspoon onion powder

½ teaspoon garlic powder

2 teaspoons poppy seeds

1 tablespoon sesame seeds

1. Preheat the oven to 350°F.

2. In a medium mixing bowl, add the ground flaxseeds, salt, and optional spices and stir with a fork to evenly distribute the seasonings.

3. Add in the water, olive oil, and vinegar and stir until a dough forms. Using your hands, form the dough into a ball. It will feel slightly sticky, and that's okay, but if it seems too wet to form into a ball, allow it to sit for 10 minutes and then knead it again.

4. Place the ball of dough in the middle of a piece of parchment paper that is roughly the size of a baking sheet. Top the dough with another piece of parchment paper. Using a rolling pin, roll the dough into a thin, even layer the same size as the baking sheet.

5. Remove the top layer of parchment.

6. Using a pizza cutter, score the dough into squares or rectangles, as desired.

7. Transfer the parchment paper with the scored dough onto a baking sheet and bake for 15 minutes.

8. Using a spatula, flip the crackers over.

9. Sprinkle with a small pinch of additional sea salt, if desired.

10. Bake for another 10 to 20 minutes or until golden brown and crispy.

11. Allow to cool completely and transfer to an airtight container for storage for up to 2 weeks.

NUTRITION FACTS PER SERVING: Calories 70 Total Fat 5g Protein 3g
Total Carbohydrate 5g Dietary Fiber 4g Total Sugars 0g Added Sugars 0g

All-Seasons Fruit Crumble

SERVES 8

This crumble is a great way to turn ripe, seasonal fruit into a beautiful dessert. Most crumble or crisp recipes call for tossing the fruit with sugar and adding sugar or another sweetener to the topping. In this recipe, we rely on the natural sweetness of the fruit in the filling and blend golden raisins into the topping to sweeten it. The finely chopped raisins are barely noticeable. Because this recipe has no added sugar and is high in fiber, it can also make for a good breakfast, especially if paired with plain yogurt for additional protein.

½ cup whole-grain flour of choice, such as buckwheat or spelt

½ cup golden raisins

½ cup raw nuts, such as almonds, walnuts, or pecans (or dried, unsweetened coconut)

½ teaspoon salt

½ teaspoon cinnamon or ground ginger (optional)

¼ teaspoon other warm spice such as nutmeg or cardamom (optional)

6 tablespoons unsalted butter, cold, or 4 tablespoons coconut oil

5 cups thinly sliced fresh, sweet, seasonal fruit such as apples, pears, peaches, nectarines, or whole berries of choice. Be sure to leave the skin on the fruit to retain the fiber. If the berries are tart, try combining them with another fruit. (5 cups is around 8 small peaches, 5 medium apples, or 4 medium pears.)

1. Preheat the oven to 350°F.

2. Put the flour, raisins, nuts, salt, and spices into the food processor and process until the raisins and nuts are chopped finely.

3. Cut the cold butter into chunks, add it to the food processor, and pulse it a few times until the butter is cut into small, uniform pieces that resemble pebbles.

4. Put the fruit mixture into an unbuttered baking dish, 9-inch round or square, 2 inches deep.

5. Spread the topping evenly over the fruit.

6. Cover with foil and bake for 35 to 40 minutes. The fruit should be bubbling.

7. Uncover and bake 8 to 15 minutes more or until the topping is browned.

8. Allow to cool slightly and serve.

9. Refrigerate any leftovers. This also tastes great cold.

VARIATIONS:

Dairy-free/vegan version: Replace the 6 tablespoons butter with 4 tablespoons coconut oil.

Nut-free version: Replace the nuts with dried, unsweetened coconut.

Gluten-free version: Use buckwheat flour or gluten-free all-purpose flour.

NUTRITION FACTS PER SERVING: Calories 250 Total Fat 16g Protein 4g
Total Carbohydrate 25g Dietary Fiber 4g Total Sugars 15g Added Sugars 0g

*NOTE: recipe analyzed with peaches and almonds.

Sicilian Almond Cookies

MAKES AROUND 48 SMALL COOKIES

Looking for a beautiful holiday cookie that tastes like a treat but will leave you and your kids feeling good, even hours after you eat it? The only sweetener used in this recipe is dates, which also adds fiber and other nutrients. The almond flour, which makes the basis of the dough, and the pistachios used for the coating contribute additional fiber as well as protein and healthy fats. The egg whites add protein as well. In addition to being nutritious, these cookies are beautifully festive—the pistachio and cherry version looks like little holiday wreaths.

Note: When developing this recipe, I used a recipe from David Lebovitz's blog as a starting point but made a number of modifications.

Dough:

3 cups almond flour

Generous pinch of salt

2 cups pitted, unsweetened dates

⅓ cup water

5 egg whites (3 for the dough and 2 for the coating) at room temperature

Toppings:

1 cup unsalted, raw pistachios, chopped (can also use pine nuts or sliced almonds)

48 dried, unsweetened cherries (roughly ½ cup if small) (can also use quartered dried apricots)

Maldon salt or other high-quality sea salt, for sprinkling

1. Preheat the oven to 325°F.

2. Cover a baking sheet with parchment paper.

3. In a small bowl, combine the almond flour and the salt and set aside.

4. In a food processor (or chopper), blend the dates and the water into a creamy paste. It is okay if there are still small, visible bits of dates in the paste.

5. Separate the egg whites from the yolks. Crack 3 into a medium bowl for beating and 2 into a small bowl that you will use to coat the cookies. (You won't need the yolks for this recipe.)

6. Beat the 3 egg whites until soft peaks form.

7. Using a rubber scraper, fold the date paste into the whites. This will deflate them some and that is okay.

8. Fold in the dry ingredients and continue blending until a dough forms in the middle of the bowl. It is okay if it feels sticky/gooey.

9. Shape the dough into small balls, slightly smaller than 1 inch each. This should make around 48.

10. Using a fork, stir the remaining 2 egg whites to loosen them up. Chop your pistachios if you haven't already and put them in another bowl.

11. Dip each of the balls into the egg white and then roll in the pistachios (or other nuts).

12. Flatten each ball into a small disk and coat with additional nuts, if needed.

13. Create an indent in each cookie and top with a dried cherry (or apricot piece).

14. Sprinkle a tiny amount of sea salt on top of each cookie.

15. Place on the baking sheet.

16. Bake the cookies for about 25 minutes or until they are golden brown. For even browning, it is helpful to rotate the pan around mid-baking.

17. Allow to cool for a few minutes before transferring them from the baking sheet.

NUTRITION FACTS PER SERVING (1 COOKIE): Calories 70 Total Fat 4g Protein 2g Total Carbohydrate 8g Dietary Fiber 1g Total Sugars 5g Added Sugars 0g

No-Bake Chocolate Sesame Squares

MAKES 24 SQUARES

This is a great recipe for easy lunch box treats. The squares have a nice fudgy texture and flavor. Though they do not require baking, the tahini (roasted sesame seed butter) makes them taste like they have been in the oven. The balance of healthy fat and protein from the sesame seeds and tahini with the natural sweetness of the dates makes these bars a very satisfying, healthy treat.

¾ cup sesame seeds (black or white), plus 2 teaspoons for sprinkling on top, if desired

⅓ cup tahini (roasted sesame seed butter)

1½ cups unsweetened dates, pitted (around 8 oz. without pits)

½ cup rolled oats

⅓ cup unsweetened cocoa powder

2 tablespoons water, plus 1 or 2 extra tablespoons if needed

Pinch of salt

1. Combine ¾ cup sesame seeds, the tahini, dates, oats, cocoa powder, 2 tablespoons water, and salt in the bowl of a food processor. Pulse until the dates and oats become uniformly chopped and all of the other ingredients are blended. The mixture should start to pull away from the sides of the food processor and collect toward the center. Try pinching it, and if it remains too crumbly to press into a dough, add an extra tablespoon of water and continue to blend until the mixture comes together. (The amount of water needed will depend on the softness of the dates you use.)

2. Line an 8x8-inch baking pan with parchment paper or wax paper, allowing for at least 2 inches of paper to hang over on two of the sides. If you don't have parchment paper, you can press the mixture directly into the pan. Using the parchment paper allows you to be able to lift the pressed mixture out of the pan and cut it on a cutting board, which makes for neater squares. But you can also successfully slice these bars directly in the pan.

3. Put the mixture into the lined pan and cover with another sheet of parchment paper of the same size. Press down on top of the paper, pushing the mixture out toward the sides of the pan, creating a uniformly thick layer. You can use something flat, like the bottom of a measuring cup, to help flatten and smooth the mixture.

4. Sprinkle the 2 teaspoons of sesame seeds over the top if desired.

5. Put the pan into the refrigerator and chill for at least 30 minutes. Lift the pressed mixture out of the pan using the sides of the paper. Transfer to a cutting board and slice into 2x2-inch squares. Any scraps can be rolled into balls, like energy bites.

6. Store in the refrigerator for up to 1 week or freeze the cut squares for up to 3 months.

NUTRITION FACTS PER SERVING (1 SQUARE): Calories 70 Total Fat 3.5g Protein 2g Total Carbohydrate 10g Dietary Fiber 2g Total Sugars 6g Added Sugars 0g

Whole Fruit Pops

MAKES 4 TO 6 POPS, DEPENDING ON THE SIZE OF THE MOLDS USED

Even the healthier-seeming Popsicles sold at the store usually contain juice and/or added sugar and not whole fruit. These pops are so easy to make, and because you use blended whole fruit, you retain the natural fiber. We like silicone molds that lie horizontal for freezing and use wooden Popsicle sticks. They are very easy to unmold, and you can easily layer in different fruit purees for rainbow pops.

2 cups cut, juicy, seasonal fresh fruit, such as cubed melon, pineapple, mango, strawberries, kiwi, or peach

Additional fruits like blueberries or raspberries for decoration (optional)

1. Place the cut fruit in a chopper, food processor, or blender. Process until liquefied. Some small chunks are okay, too.

2. Spoon the pureed fruit into Popsicle molds (or paper cups), drop in any extra fruits for decoration if using, and add sticks. If using horizontal molds, put the sticks in first and then spoon in the puree, adding multiple fruits side by side if desired.

3. Freeze until solid.

4. Unmold and enjoy.

VARIATIONS:

Add plain yogurt, coconut milk, or other milk of choice for creamy pops.

For a refreshing twist, add a squeeze of fresh lime juice to your fruit puree. We especially like this with watermelon.

For homemade fudgesicles, blend 1 banana with ⅓ cup almond milk and 2 teaspoons of cocoa powder.

NUTRITION FACTS PER SERVING: Calories 35 **Total Fat** 0g **Protein** 0g **Total Carbohydrate** 9g **Dietary Fiber** 1g **Total Sugars** 7g **Added Sugars** 0g

*NOTE: recipe analyzed for pineapple pops.

Zesty Orange and Pistachio Cake

SERVES 12

This cake has a vibrant, bright flavor and color thanks to the use of blended whole oranges, peel and all. The pistachios make for a perfect contrast to the orange. You can also use the batter to make cupcakes, which are fun for birthdays and other special occasions. Because this cake is high in fiber and protein, it is much less likely to give party guests a sugar rush than a standard cake.

Note: A Paleo Orange Cake recipe from Elana's Pantry was used as inspiration for this cake.

Cooking oil or spray of choice, for greasing the pan

2 small to medium oranges, preferably unwaxed, around 6 oz. each

4 large eggs

1 teaspoon vanilla extract

1¼ cups pitted dates

⅓ cup raw, shelled pistachios, plus 1 tablespoon for topping

½ teaspoon salt

½ teaspoon baking soda

2½ cups almond flour

1. Preheat the oven to 350°F.

2. Line the bottom of a 9-inch springform pan with parchment paper cut into a circle of the same size and grease the sides of the pan with cooking spray or oil of choice.

3. Put the oranges in a saucepan and cover with water. Bring to a boil and simmer for 20 minutes to soften the peels. (If you are not sure if the oranges are waxed, scrub them before boiling.)

4. Cool the oranges and put them whole (peels included) in a high-speed blender or food processor (halve them if necessary to allow them to fit).

5. Add the eggs and vanilla and blend until the orange peels are evenly chopped.

6. Add the dates and ⅓ cup pistachios and blend until you have a uniform-looking texture.

7. Add the salt, baking soda, and almond flour and blend until incorporated.

recipe continues

You may need to scrape down the sides of the blender to push the almond flour down and blend again.

8. Using a spatula, transfer the batter to the pan, smoothing it out into an even layer.

9. Sprinkle the 1 tablespoon of pistachios on top, pressing them lightly into the batter to anchor them and prevent them from burning.

10. Bake for 35 to 40 minutes or until golden brown and a toothpick inserted into the middle of the cake comes out clean.

11. Allow to cool in the pan for at least an hour, run a butter knife around the sides of the pan, and then unmold and serve.

NUTRITION FACTS PER SERVING: Total Fat 13g Protein 7g Total Carbohydrate 18g Dietary Fiber 4g Total Sugars 12g Added Sugars 0g

Chocolate Hazelnut Pear Cake

SERVES 12

Topped with pear slices, this cake is a gorgeous dessert for special occasions. The batter also works nicely as cupcakes/muffins.

Cooking spray or the oil of your choice, to grease the pan

1¼ cups raw hazelnuts

1 cup rolled oats (not instant)

½ teaspoon salt

½ teaspoon baking soda

3 medium ripe pears, approximately 7 oz. each (two for the cake and one for the topping)

4 large eggs

⅓ cup unsweetened cocoa powder

1 teaspoon vanilla extract

1 cup dates

1. Preheat the oven to 350°F.

2. Line the bottom of a 9-inch springform pan with parchment paper cut into a circle of the same size.

3. Spray the sides of the pan with cooking spray, or lightly grease with an oil of choice.

4. Put the hazelnuts in the bowl of a food processor and grind them until they resemble a coarse flour.

5. Add the oats, salt, and baking soda and process until evenly ground.

6. Wash the pears. Remove the stems and cores from two of them (leaving the skin on) and add them to the food processor. Reserve the other pear.

7. Add the eggs, cocoa powder, vanilla, and dates to the food processor along with two of the pears and process until smooth.

8. Pour the batter into the prepared cake pan.

9. Cut the remaining pear for the topping: cut off the stem and base and then slice it in quarters lengthwise, leaving the skin on. Remove the core and then slice each quarter thinly lengthwise. Top the cake with the pear slices, arranging them with slices starting at the middle and reaching to the edge of the pan, fanning around in a circular pattern.

10. Bake the cake in the middle of the oven for 50 to 60 minutes or until a toothpick inserted in the middle comes out clean.

NUTRITION FACTS PER SERVING: Calories 210 **Total Fat** 10g **Protein** 5g
Total Carbohydrate 26g **Dietary Fiber** 5g **Total Sugars** 14g **Added Sugars** 0g

Homemade Chocolate Milk

SERVES 1

Many parents feel that the pros of chocolate milk outweigh the cons and are fine with letting their kids have it. If it takes extra sugar to help kids get more calcium, they reason, then so be it. However, chocolate milk typically has double the amount of sugar as plain milk. If your kids like chocolate milk, you don't have to settle for a product that has added sugar and processed ingredients. Try this flexible recipe to make a chocolate milk drink at home without added sugars that is customized to your child's preferences. If you use a quarter of a banana as a natural sweetener, one serving has 15 grams of sugar, none of which is added sugar. The banana also provides extra nutrients and fiber.

1 cup unsweetened milk of choice (regular or nut milk)

½ cup ice (optional)

1 teaspoon unsweetened cocoa powder, raw cacao powder, or cacao nibs

Whole fruit sweetener: ¼ to ½ of a ripe banana or 1 to 2 dates (or a combination)

Optional additions: 2 teaspoons additional protein/healthy fat, such as nut butter, nuts, or unsweetened protein powder of choice

Optional toppings: chopped nuts, fruits, cacao nibs, or cacao/cocoa powder

1. Put the milk, ice if desired, cocoa powder, fruit sweetener, and additional protein if desired in a blender and blend until smooth.

2. Pour into a cup or a shallow bowl for sipping or eating with a spoon.

3. Sprinkle with optional toppings and serve.

NUTRITION FACTS PER SERVING: Calories 180 Total Fat 8g Protein 9g Total Carbohydrate 20g Dietary Fiber 1g Total Sugars 15g Added Sugars 0g

*NOTE: nutrition facts generated using whole milk with ¼ banana as a sweetener.

Sunshine Smoothie

SERVES 4

Here is a nice alternative to orange juice for a breakfast drink or a refreshing afternoon treat. By blending the entire (peeled) orange, you retain the natural fiber of the pulp.

1 medium orange

1 cup fresh or frozen peach slices

1 cup fresh or frozen pineapple chunks

½ to 1 cup ice (optional)

1. Cut the peel off the orange and quarter it.

2. Put the orange, peach slices, pineapple chunks, and ice if desired in a blender and blend until smooth.

3. Pour into glasses and serve. This can also be served in a bowl with a spoon, if desired.

VARIATIONS:

Zest the orange before you peel it and add the zest to the smoothie for a stronger orange flavor.

Substitute fresh or frozen mango for the peaches or the pineapple.

Top with bee pollen, orange zest, thinly sliced kumquats, or chopped almonds.

Add unsweetened protein powder of choice or plain yogurt to turn this into a more complete breakfast.

NUTRITION FACTS PER SERVING: Calories 50 Total Fat 0g Protein 1g
Total Carbohydrate 13g Dietary Fiber 2g Total Sugars 10g Added Sugars 0g

Basic Sugarproof Pasta and Pizza Sauce

YIELDS ABOUT 2½ CUPS

So many of the commercially available pasta and pizza sauces are full of added sugar. It's very easy to make your own version, starting with Italian "passata," which are tomatoes that have been cooked, deseeded, strained, and blended. You can make a big batch of this and freeze it in portions to use whenever you want to make pasta or pizza. You can also use this sauce as an easy base for making a simple shakshuka, or eggs poached in tomato sauce.

2 tablespoons olive oil

1 clove garlic

500g (about 18 oz.) Italian strained tomatoes (passata) or substitute canned crushed tomatoes or other canned tomatoes of choice

3 fresh basil leaves or 1 pinch dried

½ teaspoon salt

1. Put the olive oil in a small saucepan over low heat.

2. Peel the garlic and smash it with the side of a knife.

3. Add it to the saucepan and allow it to warm until you begin to smell the fragrance.

4. Add the tomatoes, basil, and salt, stirring to combine.

5. Raise the heat, bring to a boil, and then reduce the heat to a simmer.

6. Simmer for 10 to 15 minutes to allow the flavors to combine.

7. Remove the garlic and the whole basil leaves, if using fresh.

8. Store in the refrigerator for up to 1 week or freeze in portions to use in the future.

NUTRITION FACTS PER SERVING (¼ CUP): Calories 15 Total Fat 0g Protein 1g Total Carbohydrate 3g Dietary Fiber 1g Total Sugars 2g Added Sugars 0g

Tangerine Teriyaki Marinade/Sauce

YIELDS ¾ CUP

A teriyaki bowl can easily have the same amount of sugar as a can of soda. Use this easy Sugarproof sauce, which has no added sugar, as a healthier alternative for meals made at home. You can use it as a marinade for meats (like chicken, pork, or beef), for fish (like salmon), or for tofu. Ideally, pour the marinade over the meat/fish/tofu and allow to sit for at least ½ hour or even overnight. If time does not allow, you can spoon this sauce over the meat or fish (without marinating) and broil it, or grill it, basting with additional sauce as you go. Or you can use this as a sauce for a quick stir-fry in a wok. A small bullet attachment for a blender works great with this recipe. If you have a regular blender, consider doubling the quantities to make it easier to blend.

¼ cup soy sauce or tamari

1 seedless tangerine, clementine, or satsuma, peeled

1 date

1 teaspoon sesame oil

1 slice fresh ginger, peeled (about 1 teaspoon) (optional)

1. Add the soy sauce, tangerine, date, sesame oil, and ginger to a blender or a mini food processor.

2. Blend until liquefied and the date and ginger are well integrated. And that's it!

Note: If you can't find a tangerine, you can substitute half an orange. Peel the orange and remove any seeds before adding to the blender.

NUTRITION FACTS PER SERVING (1 TABLESPOON): Calories 15 Total Fat 0.5g Protein 1g Total Carbohydrate 2g Dietary Fiber 0g Total Sugars 1g Added Sugars 0g

Super Green Sauce

YIELDS 1 CUP

If your kids are big fans of ketchup or barbecue sauce, which are very high in sugar, introducing this sauce is a great way to expand their tastes and skip some sugar in the process. It is like a variation of Italian salsa verde, which is typically served with meat. But once you and your kids get into this sauce, you will likely find yourself starting to put it on everything, from meat to roasted potatoes, to sandwiches, to scrambled eggs, to soups, to grain bowl meals. Even very young kids can help prepare the sauce by washing the parsley, helping spin it dry, and picking the leaves off the stems. Older kids who can use the blender or food processor can make the entire sauce themselves.

2 cups flat-leaf parsley leaves, packed (about the amount from 1 large or 2 small bunches)

⅔ cup olive oil, plus more if needed

Zest from 1 lemon (optional)

A generous squeeze of fresh lemon juice (optional)

1 tablespoon capers, rinsed and drained

1 clove garlic

½ teaspoon salt

1. Wash the parsley and dry it with a salad spinner or a clean kitchen towel. Remove and discard the large stems (some smaller ones are okay to leave).

2. Put the parsley, olive oil, lemon zest if using, lemon juice if desired, capers, garlic, and salt in a food processor or blender and blend until you have a relatively uniformly textured sauce. If it is not blending easily, add some extra oil.

3. Transfer to a small serving dish and enjoy with meat, vegetables, eggs, sandwiches, or pasta salad. It will keep for up to 5 days in the refrigerator.

Note: This sauce can also be made by hand by chopping the parsley, capers, and garlic on a cutting board with a knife, putting them in a small bowl, and stirring in the other ingredients.

Variations:
Try the sauce with other herbs/greens such as cilantro or arugula, or a mixture of herbs, to create different flavor profiles.

NUTRITION FACTS PER SERVING (1 TABLESPOON): **Calories** 80 **Total Fat** 9g **Protein** 0g **Total Carbohydrate** 1g **Dietary Fiber** 0g **Total Sugars** 0g **Added Sugars** 0g

Simple Fruit Compotes

YIELDS AROUND 1 CUP

Fruit compotes can easily be made with no added sugar and are a great alternative to jam or jelly for toast. They also make a good substitute for honey or maple syrup and add natural sweetness to plain yogurt, oatmeal, pancakes, or crepes. You can use many different fruits to make them. Two of our favorites are the blueberry and apple/pear versions we show here. We like to keep the blueberry version very simple. For the apple/pear versions, we especially like apple with raisin and cinnamon and pear with vanilla and lemon zest. You can make a double batch and keep these in the refrigerator for up to a week.

Pure Blueberry   3 tablespoons water (optional)

3 cups fresh or frozen blueberries

1. If using fresh blueberries, rinse and drain them.

2. Put the berries in a small saucepan and begin to warm them slowly on low heat. If using fresh blueberries, you can add a few tablespoons of water to prevent them from sticking to the pan. If using frozen, you are not likely to need any liquid. As they begin to warm, smash them with a fork to release their juice. Simmer for 5 to 10 minutes, stirring occasionally, until they begin to look jammy in consistency. Turn off the heat and you will notice that the compote thickens more as it cools. Serve immediately or store in the refrigerator for up to 1 week.

NUTRITION FACTS PER SERVING (2 TABLESPOONS): Calories 30 Total Fat 0g
Protein 0g Total Carbohydrate 8g Dietary Fiber 1g Total Sugars 6g Added Sugars 0g

recipe continues

Apple/Pear Compote

2 medium apples or pears

1 cup water

Optional flavorings:

2 tablespoons raisins

½ teaspoon cinnamon

¼ teaspoon nutmeg

1 teaspoon grated lemon or orange zest

1 teaspoon vanilla extract

1. Wash the apples or pears but do not peel them so you retain the fiber. Thinly slice them or cut them into small cubes, removing the stem and core.

2. Add the slices or cubes to a small saucepan along with the water and add in any of the optional flavorings.

3. Bring to a boil over medium heat. Reduce the heat to low to allow the apple or pear to simmer and soften.

4. After 20 to 25 minutes, the apple or pear should be soft, the water will have evaporated, and the fruit may even begin to caramelize.

5. Turn off the heat and serve or allow it to cool and store it in the refrigerator for up to 1 week.

NUTRITION FACTS PER SERVING (2 TABLESPOONS, FOR PLAIN APPLE VERSION): Calories 25 Total Fat 0g Protein 0g Total Carbohydrate 6g Dietary Fiber 1g Total Sugars 5g Added Sugars 0g

Acknowledgments

We are extremely grateful to our agent, Betsy Amster, who saw the potential value of *Sugarproof* and whose guidance was invaluable in helping us shape the material to bring it to a broad audience. We are also extremely grateful to our consulting editor, Leigh Ann Hirschman, whose inspired ideas, including the title of the book, helped bring our scientific writing to life. We are grateful to Lucia Watson and her team at Avery for also believing in this project and giving us the opportunity to publish this book. We are grateful to several colleagues who helped review some of the scientific content, including Donna Spruijt-Metz, who helped shape Chapter 6, Kimber Stanhope who reviewed the scientific content in Part 1, Allison Sylvetsky for always being so generous in sharing her wide knowledge on the topic of low-calorie sweeteners, and Nicole Avena for her expertise on the effects of sugar on the brain. Thank you to the many families who helped us test our 7 Day and 28-Day Challenges. The feedback you provided on our materials and recipes was invaluable. And the stories you shared with us about your experiences were key in bringing this book to life.

Michael's Personal Acknowledgment

I am extremely grateful to all of my colleagues and collaborators that I have had the good fortune to work with over the years, not just at USC and Children's Hospital Los Angeles but also many amazing people around the world whom I have had the good fortune to interact with over the past three decades. Our interactions and discussions have helped in immeasurable ways to shape my thinking and move the science forward. My clinical research in children would also not be possible without an incredible group of pediatric specialists whom I have worked with over the years. This group includes Marc Weigensberg, Rohit Kohli, Jennifer Raymond, Juan Espinoza, Alaina Vidmar, Brad Peterson, and Frank Sinatra, who gave me a better understanding of fatty liver disease in children. To the amazing students and fellows I have worked with over the years, too many to mention here but who have all contributed to the progression of our research together. Many have specifically contributed to our work with sugar and spent endless hours doing studies, poring over the data, and writing manuscripts that have helped shift the field of sugar and child health forward: Jaimie Davis, Courtney Byrd-Williams, Rebecca Hasson, Tanja Adam, Kim-Anne Le, Ryan Walker, Claudia Toledo-Corral, Brandon Kayser, Lauren Gyllenhammer, Tanya Alderete, Emily Noble, Jasmine Plows, Paige Berger, and Roshonda Jones. Thank you to all of my students and trainees over the years for responding to my constant pleas to *"show me the data!"* and for your passion and dedication. Mentoring you and watching you evolve has been the most memorable part of this career. Thank you also to the many dedicated and passionate research assistants, coordinators, dieticians, and other staff who have worked with me over the years to organize and implement the studies to make the research possible. Finally, a big thanks to all the families and children who have participated in our research studies and dedicated their time and effort in the name of nutrition science. We literally couldn't have done all this work without you.

To my mum, who introduced me to cooking at a young age, and for teaching me to *"say it like it is."*

I'm extremely grateful to Lori. I couldn't have asked for a better person to spend my adult life with, or for a better proofreader who always asks probing questions that lead me to dig deeper. Lastly to my amazing daughters, Coco and Orla. You bring me such joy and you help keep me young—even though you have watched me go gray. You and your generation bring me such hope for the future through your insistence on unity, inclusiveness, and civility in this world.

Emily's Personal Acknowledgment

First and foremost I would like to thank Michael for inviting me to work with him on this project. It's been rewarding and energizing for me, even despite the late nights and early mornings of passing drafts back and forth across time zones between the United States and the UK. Also thank you to other professional mentors, including Jaimie, Lourdes, Donna, and Jean, who trained me in health behavior research. As far as my culinary education goes, I'm especially grateful for Alice, Esther, Greg, Lili, and Paolo. Each of you has shown me that the most important ingredient in any dish is your desire to make it. Also, the end result of what you make is only as good as the quality of the ingredients you start with. Simply put: source good ingredients and put enthusiasm and love into preparing them, and the end result will be delicious.

Without the support of my family and friends, I would not have been able to successfully dedicate myself to this project, especially in the wake of my husband's death. Thank you for being there with me either in person or in spirit as I went through all the waves of grief over this last year while trying to write.

Mom and Dad, you have given me everything, and the way that you have mobilized to help me in this particular time of need has been especially touching. Thank you for all the love and joy you give to me and the boys. Leo and Alex, you keep me smiling and I'm lucky to be your mommy/mamma/mum. Here's to more dance parties in the kitchen. I'm also immensely grateful for other family, including Laird, Kim, Lynna, Lisa, Helen and Anthony, Tom, Beth and Brian, John and Trish, and Barb for your continual support. Thank you as well to Lili and Ramiro, Maria, Bernarda, Sofia, Emily F, and my whole Ecuadorian/German family as well as to Paolo and Margherita in Italy for adopting me into your families.

My tribe of friends rallied for me as well, encouraging me as I wrote. Thank you to my best friend, Emily N, for being my constant go-to for pep talks, laughs, and inspiration for keeping fit and keeping my act together in general. And thank you to your whole family, including Lloyd, Evelyn, Matt, Marc, and Meredith who have always been there for me. This book was also made better by so many of my other friends who supported me, including Sarah P, Emma A, Mindy, Jackie M, Tatiana, Katie D, Liz, Jai, Cassie, Wyatt, Elizabeth Z, Jacqueline, Lindsay, Chrissy, Jen, Helen B, Jenelle, Salva, Samer, Kat, Claudia, Rosa, Laura S, Kim-Anne, Anna, Nick, Amy, Vince, Lisa, Tracy, Taylor, Jadenne, Nadia, Stefano F, Silvia S, Vincenzo, Marco, Giovanna, Davide, Jackie B, Ulrik, Claire, Giacomo, Eloisa, Julie, Maria-Carmela, Santo, Maria-Letizia, Gianni, Ilaria,

Michaela, Letizia G, Cinzia, Maiju, Adrianna, Silvia T, Stefano C, Mon, Bex, Deirdre, Roisin, Lidia, Lucy, Isabella, Katie M, Tito, Sinead, Gavin, Becki, Matt, Sadie, Jenny W, Mark, and Ravi.

Thank you to everyone who helped test our recipes and suggestions, including Silvia T, Nadia, Junko, E'lain, Scarlet, Sarah M, Marla, Theresa, Deirdre, Sinead, Laura O'B, Emma T, Katie M, Kate, Jemma, Gemma, Nichola, Brenda, Amy, Anna, Judy, Shannon, Danielle, Emma A, Emily N, Liz, Jenelle, Tammy, Chrissy, Ace, Georgiana, Ruby, Jenny S, Suzanna, Kelley, Cheli, Leah, Lauren, Anita, Yuliya, Abby, Kristen, Megan, Cathy, Jessica, and Melissa. A special thanks (and apology) to anyone who tried the first round of muffins.

I'm deeply grateful for all of you who helped me during this last year, which has been the hardest year of my life so far, but also the one that I have learned and grown the most in.

Index

About the Authors

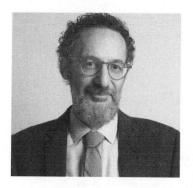

Michael I. Goran, PhD, is one of the world's most widely recognized experts in childhood nutrition and obesity research, with more than thirty years of experience as a researcher, mentor, and educator. He is a Professor of Pediatrics at the University of Southern California, Keck School of Medicine; Co-Director of the USC Diabetes and Obesity Research Institute; and leads the Program in Diabetes and Obesity at Children's Hospital Los Angeles. He holds the Dr. Robert C. and Veronica Atkins Endowed Chair in Childhood Obesity and Diabetes. Michael is a native of Glasgow, Scotland, and received his PhD from the University of Manchester, UK.

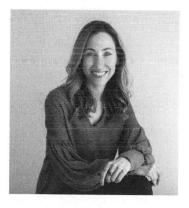

Emily E. Ventura, PhD, MPH, is an experienced nutrition educator, public health advocate, writer, and cook. She completed her master's in public health and PhD in health behavior research at the University of Southern California. She was selected as a Fulbright Scholar to teach Public Health Nutrition in Italy and is a mother to two young boys.

Photographs of the authors by Lori Lovoy-Goran and Dorte Kjaerulff